Renal Diet
2 in 1

Renal Diet and Cookbook.

The Ultimate Guide

With Low Sodium, Potassium and Phosphorus.

Includes 100 Healthy Recipes

and 21 Days Meal Plan

SUSAN SIMON

mentioned are done without written consent and can in no way be considered an endorsement from the trademark holder.

Table of Contents

RENAL DIET

Introduction 1

Chapter 1: Kidney Disease 5

Chapter 2: Symptoms and Causes of Kidney Disease 16

Chapter 3: Introduction to Renal Diet 21

Chapter 4: Benefits of Renal Diet 31

Chapter 5: How to Limit Sodium, Potassium And Phosphorus In The Diet 34

Chapter 6: What You Can Eat and What You Can Avoid in Renal Diet 44

Chapter 7: Top 10 Foods to Eat for Kidney Health 64

Chapter 8: Renal Diet Meal Plan 73

Chapter 9: How to Slow Kidney Disease 78

Chapter 10: The Reasons Diets Don't Work 84

Chapter 11: The Basics of Renal Diet 92

Chapter 12: Eating Well To Live Well 99

Chapter 13: Pointers to Remember When Slow Cooking 105

Conclusion 110

RENAL DIET COOKBOOK

Introduction 115

Chapeter 1: Introduction to Renal Diet 117

Chapeter 2: Benefits of Renal Diet 126

Chapter 3: What You Can Eat And What You Can Avoid In Renal Diet 128

Chapter 4: Breakfast Recipes 131

Chapter 5: Lunch Recipes   152

Chapter 6: Dinner Recipes   172

Chapter 7: Dessert Recipe   199

Chapter 8 : 21-Day Kidney Diet Plan   223

Chapter 9: Getting Used to Low-Sodium Diet Regimen   233

Chapter 10: Renal Diet And Lifestyle Guidance   241

Conclusion   250

Renal Diet

Diet Plan and Nutrition Guide

With Low Sodium,

Potassium and Phosphorus

Meal Plan Solution

SUSAN SIMON

Introduction

You might be wondering what really constitutes the renal diet. Kidney sufferers are more concerned about what they CAN eat than what they CAN'T eat.

A diet can be healthy and effective for one person, while it may not be so-effective to another person, totally forgetting the fact that some food has a negative effect on the kidneys.

The following are renal diet tips that every kidney patient should bear in mind:

1.   Know what you can only eat – the following list of food is deemed to be healthy for your kidneys:

   a.   Fruits – such as apples, peach, grapes, apricot, blueberries, strawberries, pineapple, raspberries, and watermelon.

   b.   Vegetables – like cauliflower, garlic, onion, mung beans, cabbage, and asparagus.

   c.   Protein – such as tofu, chicken, and fish.

   d.   Herbs and spices - like curry powder, sesame seeds, olive oil, oregano, and paprika.

2.   Avoid food that is bad for the kidneys. Some of them include:

   a.   Alcohol – with the exemption that it is done in moderation and checked with one's doctor. For women, the safe levels of drinking are 1 drink per day. For men, two drinks per day are allowed.

   b.   Sugar

   c.   Processed food

   d.   Red meat

   e.   Food with gluten – this includes rye, spelt, and kamut. The safest grain alternatives are quinoa, rice, millet, amaranth, buckwheat, and teff.

f.   Patients with kidney disease should avoid food high in sodium and phosphorus. Some of the examples include muffins, waffles, cookies, biscuits, pancakes, pretzels, frozen food, soy sauce, seasoned salt, and other condiments.

3.   Monitor your consumption of sodium, potassium, protein, and phosphorus – make sure that they are within the healthy limits. Unfortunately, healthy limits would depend on the level or stage of kidney disease a person has. This is why it is important that you consult a nutritionist so a proper renal diet can be customized just for you. Also, have your blood tested so you'll know which nutrients are low or high so you may easily alter your diet accordingly.

4.   Hydrate your body with the "right" fluids - this means no coffee, alcohol, caffeinated beverages, soda pop, tea, soft drinks, and even those labeled with "sugar-free' drinks. It is best to consume more water, herbal teas such as lemon, green tea, ginger, berries, and fresh vegetable/fruit juices.

5.   Dedication is a must – if you want to reverse your condition and improve your kidney function, you must follow the renal diet to the letter. According to research, a single slip; this means a single cheat meal would mean undoing all the good work that you have started. Therefore, the renal diet needs to be followed religiously. It should be second nature to you, a kind of lifestyle, and a part of you. With dedication and consistency, all the hard work will soon pay off especially when you see your creatinine levels drop.

6.   If you can follow a whole, unprocessed, renal diet, then meal times won't be a burden. Soon, you will reap the benefits of having healthier kidneys.

The Basics of the Renal Diet

People who suffer from kidney diseases specifically need to monitor their potassium, sodium, and phosphorus intakes. Certain ingredients need to be controlled:

Sodium

This is generally found in salt and is mostly used as a seasoning in food. However, if you are on a renal diet, it is a must that sodium is reduced through the following:

- Do not use salt as a seasoning when cooking food
- Do not put salt directly to your food.
- Say no to processed food as they contain too much sodium such as hotdogs, sausage, ham, canned soup, nuggets, and more.
- Make it a habit to always read the labels. If you are going to buy canned vegetables, always go for the label that says "no salt added".

According to studies, children and adult are advised to consume 2,300mg of sodium a day. But, if you have kidney disease, it is recommended that you reduce it to 1,500mg or lower per day.

Potassium

This is another important nutrient but should be minimized or not taken at all when you have kidney disease. This is because potassium could build up in the blood and could cause irregular heartbeat, or worse, heart attack. Potassium is usually found in bananas, oranges, prunes, melons, squash, Swiss chard, pumpkin, and kale. Potatoes and sweet potatoes should be eaten in small amounts.

The recommended potassium for people with kidney problems is less than 2,000 mg a day.

Phosphorus

This is another mineral that can build up in the blood especially when the kidneys do not work properly. When this happens, bone disease can become a problem. Some of the food to avoid or limit include:

- Limit milk intake to 1 cup a day.
- Limit consumption of veggies rich in phosphorus to 1 cup a week. Some of them include broccoli, Brussels sprouts, dried beans, and mushrooms.
- Cereals should also be limited to 1 serving per weeks such as granola, oatmeal, bran, and wheat cereals.

The recommended phosphorus for people with kidney disease is 800 to 1,000 mg per day.

As for protein intake, the recommended intake for pre-dialysis patients is 37-41 grams per day.

Chapter 1: Kidney Disease

What is Chronic Kidney Disease (CKD)?

There is chronic kidney disease (CKD) when it is damaged kidneys or kidney function decline for three months or more. There are five stages of evolution of a CRM according to the severity of the renal involvement or the degree of deterioration of its function.

Sometimes the kidney failure suddenly occurs. In this case, it is called an acute failure of the kidney. An injury, infection, or something else may be the cause. Acute renal failure is often treated with urgency by dialysis for some time. Often, kidney function recovers itself. Generally, this disease settles slowly and silently, but it progresses over the years. People with CKD do not necessarily go from stage 1 to stage 5 of the disease. Stage 5 of the disease is known under the name of end stage renal disease (ESRD) or kidney failure in the final stage.

It is important to know that the expressions terminal, final, and ultimate mean the end of any function of the kidneys (kidneys working at less than 15% of their normal capacity) and not the end of your life. To stay alive at this stage of the disease, it is necessary to resort to dialysis or a kidney transplant. Dialysis and transplantation are known as renal replacement therapy (TRS).

This means that dialysis or the transplanted kidney will "supplement" or "replace" the sick kidneys and do their job.

What Are the Causes of Chronic Kidney Disease?

There are different kinds of diseases and disorders of the kidneys. At present, we do not know for sure all the causes. Some are hereditary, while others develop with age. They are often associated with another disease, such as diabetes, heart disease, or high blood pressure.

Most kidney diseases attack kidney filters, damaging their ability to eliminate waste and excess fluids. For the moment, no treatment can cure these diseases, but it is possible to prevent them or to slow down their evolution. This is especially true of diseases such as diabetes and hypertension, the leading causes of kidney failure.

Who Runs the Risk of Having a CKD?

Even though people with diabetes use insulin by injection or take medication, they are not able to shelter the lesion of some small blood vessels, like those in the retina of the eye. In this case, the retina may be damaged, resulting in loss of vision. Also, they are not immune to the deterioration of the fragile blood vessels of the renal filters.

Progressive deterioration of the kidneys is seen when urine tests show higher and higher protein levels. As the disease progresses, the number of protein increases. As for treatment, the sooner it starts (for example, with drugs such as ACE inhibitors or A2 blocking agents), the more likely it is to slow the progression of the disease. Kidney disease caused by diabetes can slow the evolution of the disease regardless of its stage.

Over time, diabetes can reach kidney filters at a point of no return: the kidneys no longer function, and renal replacement therapy becomes essential. People with diabetes are prone to infections, which are changing rapidly. If these infections, especially those of the urinary tract, are not treated, they can damage the kidneys. It is recommended that people with diabetes not overlook any infection and have it treated immediately.

Hypertension

The kidneys secrete a hormone that plays an important role in increasing or reducing blood pressure. When the kidneys are so affected that they do not function properly, the secretion of this hormone can increase and cause hypertension, which in turn, damages the kidneys. It is, therefore, necessary to closely monitor hypertension to avoid the deterioration of renal function in the long term.

Glomerulonephritis

The glomerulonephritis, or nephritis, declares when glomeruli, these little tiny filters used to purify the blood, deteriorates. There are several kinds of glomerulonephritis. Some are hereditary, while others occur as a result of certain diseases such as strep throat. The causes of most glomerulonephritis are not yet known. Some glomerulonephritis cure without medical treatment, while others require prescription drugs. Some do not respond to any treatment and who have chronic kidney disease. Some clues suggest that glomerulonephritis is due to a deficiency in the immune system of the body.

Autosomal Dominant Polycystic Disease

Often in their forties, people with the disease will need dialysis or kidney transplant. But because the loss of kidney function is changing at a different pace, depending on the individual, the time between the onset of cysts and the need for dialysis varies widely. Since the disease is hereditary, people are advised to inform other family members to carry out the required tests as they too may be affected.

The Obstruction of the Urinary Tract

Any obstruction (or blockage) of the urinary tract may damage the kidneys. Obstructions can occur in the ureter or at the end of the bladder. Narrowing of the ureter at the superior or inferior level is sometimes due to congenital malformations, which sometimes leads to chronic kidney disease in children. In adults, increased prostate volume, kidney stones, or tumors often obstruct the urinary tract.

Reflux Nephropathy

The reflux nephropathy is the new name of the former "chronic pyelonephritis."

Illegal Drugs

The use of illegal drugs can cause kidney damage. Over-the-counter medications (without a prescription) High-dose and long-term use of over-the-counter medications can cause kidney damage.

Important: Beware of medications, including herbal remedies, sold without a prescription. It would be wiser to seek the advice of your doctor before buying them.

Prescription Drugs

Some medications prescribed to people with kidney disease cause renal dysfunction. The lesions are sometimes reversible and sometimes irreversible. Many medications prescribed by prescription are safe but provided the doctor makes changes accurate to the dosage. So always ask your doctor or your pharmacist, information about potential side effects of prescribed drugs.

Other Kidney Disorders

Other issues can affect the kidneys, such as, for example, kidney stones, Syndrome Alport, Fabry disease, Wilms tumor (children only), not including infections of bacterial origin.

What Are the Symptoms of Kidney Disease?

In chronic kidney disease, the deterioration of kidney function is gradual. At the very beginning of the CKD, there are hardly any warning signs or apparent symptoms. In some cases, it is difficult to detect any evidence while the kidneys are already severely affected.

Laboratory analysis of proteins and blood in the urine (urine analysis) can show at an early stage whether the kidney is affected or not. The calculation of serum creatinine levels makes it possible to know, well before other signs occur, whether the kidneys function well or not, or whether there is a decrease in renal function.

Warning signs or symptoms of kidney disease:

- High blood pressure
- The swelling of the eyes, hands, and feet
- Blood in the urine, cloudy or dark urine such as tea
- The presence of proteins in the urine
- Urines foamier than normal
- The frequent urge to urinate during the night
- Less urine or difficulty urinating
- Fatigue, difficulty concentrating

- Loss of appetite or weight
- Generalized and persistent itching

The Uremia

"Uremia" is a word that comes from the Greek word meaning Urine in the blood. The uremia declares when the kidneys no longer function normally and are no longer able to remove waste from the body. Many symptoms of uremia occur when kidney function deteriorates. This varies from person to person, but in most of them, the symptoms occur when the kidneys are functioning at less than 20 - 30% of their normal capacity. The more the kidney function is degraded, the more waste accumulates in the blood.

Symptoms may worsen and may include shortness of breath, nausea, vomiting, itching, and headache. Also, high blood pressure, anemia, or increased levels of acid and potassium in the blood may cause even more serious problems. Even before the worsening of the uremia, you may be prescribed dialysis or grafting.

Warning signs or possible symptoms of uremia:

- Weight loss
- Memory problems
- Tiredness
- Leg cramps
- Weakness
- The insomnia
- Nausea
- Itches
- Vomiting
- The intolerance to cold
- A bad feeling
- Chest pain taste in the mouth
- A yellowish color or brownish skin

- Lack of appetite
- The shaking of the legs
- A decrease in sexual desire
- The shortness of breath
- Bruising tendencies

What Can Be Done to Prevent the Evolution of a CKD?

The chronic renal disease does not necessarily make it to end-stage renal failure. There are some options to help possibly prevent or even decrease the rate of your progress. By adopting healthy habits, many people with CKDs have a better quality of life. Well-being is a complete physical, mental, and social state. Ask the members of your health care team to explain how to strive for wellness and adopt principles such as:

- A well-balanced diet
- Physical activities at regular intervals (ideally 45 to 60 minutes four to five times a week)
- Well-controlled blood pressure
- Balanced blood glucose (in the presence of diabetes)
- Stop smoking
- Control of anemia (maintenance of a normal blood count)
- Maintaining a healthy weight
- Moderation in alcohol consumption (maximum of two drinks per day)
- Taking medication according to the doctor's instructions
- It is also important to be familiar with your kidney disease and to listen to the information and advice given to you from your doctor and medical care team.

Recommendations to Prevent Chronic Kidney Disease

The Ministry of Health has recommended the control of risk factors such as tobacco consumption and high cholesterol, among other measures to prevent Chronic Kidney Disease (CKD).

The health authority recalled that the lower consumption of sodium in the daily food diet, the intake of varied fruits and vegetables, as well as limiting up to five weekly servings of red and white meats, favor the protection of the kidneys and improve the quality of life. He also stressed the importance of adding at least 30 minutes of physical activity daily, not smoking and controlling blood pressure.

The people most likely to suffer from kidney disease are those with hypertension and diabetes, so it is very important to carry out controls for early diagnosis.

Chronic Kidney Disease is the alteration of the functioning of the kidneys for more than three months and the gradual loss of its functions.

The first four stages of kidney malfunction have no symptoms, so they represent a challenge by health professionals for early diagnosis to avoid Terminal Chronic Kidney Disease, which requires dialysis or transplant treatments. This last phase of the disease leads to a significant deterioration in the patient's quality of life and also has a high cost to the healthcare system.

Chronic Kidney Disease: Classification, Risk Factors, and History

Definition and Classification of Chronic Renal Disease

The CKD is defined by the presence of an anatomical and/or urinary indicator of renal impairment and/or a decrease in the rate of glomerular filtration (GFR) persisting beyond three months. This disease is classified into five stages of increasing severity, according to the GFR. The first two stages are characterized by a DFG within normal limits, require the presence of markers of renal impairment including urinary tests (proteinuria, Haematuria, or pyuria) or morphological abnormalities renal ultrasound (contours bumpy, asymmetrical in size, small kidneys or large kidneys, polycystic, etc.).

Only the other three stages are characterized by a real decrease in GFR. The end stage of chronic renal failure (CRT) or stage 5 of the CKD is defined by a GFR <15 ml/min / 1.73 m^2.

Renal impairment is defined by the presence of pathological abnormalities or biological markers of the kidney, including abnormalities of urinary or kidney morphological tests detected by imaging.

Historically, the lack of consensus in the definition of CKD (especially chronic renal failure), its severity has led to late diagnosis, inadequate medical management, and data deficiency. epidemiologically comparable at the global level.

It was not until 2002 that this gap was filled by adopting the DFG thresholds or the aforementioned CKD stages.

Risk Factors and Chronic Renal Disease

Non - modifiable risk factors, advanced age, male sex, low birth weight, race or ethnicity, genetic and hereditary factors predispose to an increased risk of CKD development. However, it must be recognized that the racial factor is sometimes difficult to analyze as it is probably associated with a genetic predisposition but also environmental and socio-economic factors such as inequalities of access to care, nutritional intake, and low birth weight.

Unmodifiable Risk Factors

- Advanced age
- Sex (masculine / feminine)
- Race / ethnicity (African Americans, Native Americans, Hispanics, Whites, African Blacks)
- Low birth weight
- Genetics / family

Modifiable Risk Factors

- Hypertension (I & P)
- Diabetes mellitus (I & P)
- Obesity (I & P)
- Proteinuria (P)
- Dyslipidemia (I & P)
- Hyperuricemia (I & P)
- Smoking (I & P)

- Alcohol consumption (I)
- Infections (I)
- Autoimmune diseases (I)
- Drug / plant poisoning / analgesic abuse (I)
- Obstructive lithiasis / uropathies (I)
- Low socio-economic class (I & P)

Abbreviations: I = initiation; P = progression.

As the main emunctory, the kidney is potentially exposed to many aggressions. Although the parenchyma has an extraordinary ability to adapt and regenerate, the CKD can progressively destroy the functional structures of the kidney: glomeruli, tubes, interstitium, and vessels. Moreover, whatever the cause or the various and multiple underlying pathophysiological mechanisms, it has a common functional consequence: chronic renal failure (CKD). This one is likely to evolve inexorably towards the terminal stage corresponding to the renal death. The latter results in serious consequences for the entire organism that has lost the constancy of the internal environment, related to uremic intoxication, on the one hand, and failures of renal, endocrine functions on the other hand.

Family history of chronic kidney disease, low birth weight, smoking and alcoholism

CKD risk factors reported elsewhere, such as HF - CKD, low birth weight, smoking, and alcoholism, did not emerge as an independent determinant of CKD. This lack of association could be explained by the difference in methodology and probably the relatively small size of the sample and the low frequency of the factors mentioned above in this work.

The frequency of HF-CKD varied between 5 and 9% according to the studies composing this dissertation. Among some subjects who knew their birth weight, they were, respectively, 3% (mass screening campaign), 6% (study in CSs), and 7% (household survey).

Concerning HF-CKD and low birth weight, lack of knowledge of the CKD and its association with HF-CKD or birth weight by both patients and the general population could partly explain this lack of association. of HF-CKD or low birth weight and the CKD.

However, low birth weight is well known, associated with a reduction in nephron mass in utero, with increased risk of diabetes mellitus, hypertension, and progressive renal impairment in adulthood. Also, the nephron deficit would increase the susceptibility of the kidneys to various assaults, such as hypertension, diabetes mellitus, and HIV infection.

In populations with low socioeconomic levels, such as those of different African or Afro-American black ethnic groups, birth weight is frequently lower. We also believe that low birth weight has not been properly researched in this work. According to several authors, the term low birth weight should not be limited to the universal birth weight threshold <2.5 Kg. For these authors, low birth weight or better, fetal hypotrophy should be defined as a small weight for the gestational age about a birth weight below the 5th or 10th percentile of weight distributions by age and sex gestation. These data were not available in this memory and can, in principle, only be correctly gathered in longitudinal studies.

As for smoking, its frequency was between 7 and 10% in the various surveys carried out in this work. In this respect, the incidence of IRT in non - diabetic subjects is multiplied by 5.9 in heavy smokers (> 15 packets/year). Another study had shown that the risk of development of albuminuria was multiplied by 3 in heavy smokers (> 20 packets/year) compared to non - smokers. The possible mechanism by which tobacco may contribute to renal impairment includes stimulation of the sympathetic nervous system, glomerular capillary hypertension, endothelial damage, and direct tubular toxicity of nicotine. The reason for the lack of association between proteinuria and smoking in all our work is unclear and requires a longitudinal study. It is possible, however, that some of the subjects studied did not admit this intoxication.

Concerning alcoholism, its frequency was respectively 28%, 20%, and 8% in the mass screening campaign, in the general population (household study) and the health structures (among the subjects at risk of alcoholism). CKD). The potential role of alcohol in the pathogenesis of the CKD remains a controversial subject. A case-control study found a significant association between IRT and consumption of> 2 glasses of alcohol/day, while another similar study did not confirm this association. Consumption of alcohol may increase the risk of CKD through initiation and/or promotion of risk factors.

Chapter 2: Symptoms and Causes of Kidney Disease

Kidneys may be small, but they do have important functions in the body. These bean-shaped organs work hard, but they may experience injuries and other problems that prevent them from functioning properly. But the question is what causes kidney disease and how to detect it?

Causes and Risk Factors

What many of us are not aware of is that the cause of kidney disease doesn't necessarily have to occur in kidneys themselves. Problems affecting our overall health and wellbeing can also induce damage to the kidneys. In the same way, common health problems can also impair the function of these organs. The most frequent causes of kidney disease are hypertension and diabetes.

High blood pressure, which affects 75 million people in the US or one in three adults, can damage blood vessels in the kidney and thereby impair their function. In other words, damage to blood vessels in the kidneys due to hypertension doesn't allow them to remove wastes and extra fluid from your body. This leads to a vicious cycle as an accumulation of waste, and extra fluid increases blood pressure. Besides damaging filtering units in kidneys, high blood pressure can also reduce the flow of blood to these organs. As you're already aware, without a blood supply, organs cannot function properly.

About 30.3 million people or 9.4% of the population in the United States have diabetes which can cause several complications. Just like hypertension, diabetes also damages small blood vessels in the kidneys. As a result, the body retains more salt and water than it should. Moreover, diabetes also causes damage to the nerves in the body, which can make it difficult for you to empty the bladder. The pressure from a full bladder can back up and damage or injure kidneys. Let's also not forget the fact that if urine remains in the body for a long time, it can lead to an infection from the fast growth of bacteria and high blood sugar levels.

Estimates show that 30% of patients with type 1 diabetes and 10% to 40% of people with type 2 diabetes will eventually experience kidney failure.

Besides diabetes and hypertension, other causes of kidney disease include:

- Infection
- Renal artery stenosis
- Heavy metal poisoning
- Lupus
- Some drugs
- Prolonged obstruction of the urinary tract from conditions such as kidney stones, enlarged prostate, some cancers

Symptoms of Kidney Disease

Signs and symptoms of kidney disease don't appear suddenly, and they develop over time. Many people don't even know they have kidney disease until it reaches late stages because they are unable to identify some warning signs. Symptoms of kidney diseases may vary from one person to another as well as their severity. But generally speaking, the most common signs of kidney disease include:

- Nausea and vomiting
- Hypertension that is difficult to control
- Loss of appetite
- Shortness of breath
- Chest pain
- Weakness or fatigue
- Sleep disturbances
- Persistent itching
- Changes in how much a patient urinates
- Swollen feet and ankles
- Reduced mental sharpness

- Muscle cramps and twitching
- Blood in urine or foamy urine

It is worth mentioning that symptoms of kidney disease can be nonspecific as they are greatly influenced by causes of these conditions and underlying diseases.

Renal Diet Overview

Kidney disease requires a proactive approach to reduce the intensity of symptoms and improve a patient's quality of life. Eating habits play a vital role in the management of kidney disease. Therefore, the most important thing you can do to manage your condition and prevent dialysis is to adopt a renal diet.

What is the Renal Diet?

A renal diet is defined as a diet that is low in protein, sodium, and phosphorus. This diet emphasizes the importance of limiting fluids and consuming high-quality proteins, but some patients may also need to decrease their intake of calcium and potassium. The main goal of the renal diet is to support kidney function and decrease the need for dialysis, but for it to work, one needs to adhere to it religiously. A renal diet is not a diet fad that comes and goes, and it's not a program one should follow for a few weeks. Instead, it's a way of life. Below you can see the breakdown of the most important components you need to monitor when on a renal diet.

Sodium

First, it's important to clarify that sodium is not a synonym for salt, as many people believe. Salt is just a compound of sodium and chloride. On the other hand, sodium is a mineral naturally present in many foods and important for body functions. In addition to potassium and chloride, sodium is an electrolyte meaning it helps control fluid levels in cells and tissues.

Sodium helps maintain blood pressure, regulates nerve function and muscle contraction, controls acid-base balance in the blood, among other things.

However, excessive levels of sodium are harmful to patients with kidney disease due to the fact these organs are unable to eliminate sodium and fluid from the body in an adequate manner.

As a result, fluid and sodium start accumulating and may cause several problems such as increased thirst, edema, hypertension, heart failure, and shortness of breath.

Phosphorus

Phosphorus is a mineral required for the maintenance and development of bones. This mineral also participates in the development of connective tissues, takes part in muscle movement, and so much more. Damaged kidneys don't remove excess phosphorus from the body. In turn, levels of this mineral accumulate and impair calcium balance, thus causing weak bones and calcium deposits in blood vessels.

Potassium

Potassium is an important mineral that participates in many functions, including muscle function, and it helps promote a healthy heartbeat. Like sodium, potassium is also necessary for fluid and electrolyte balance.

While potassium is needed for our health, patients with kidney disease do need to reduce the intake of this mineral. The reason is simple; when kidneys are damaged, they are not able to eliminate excess potassium out of the body. This causes a buildup of potassium and leads to other problems such as muscle weakness, heart attack, slow pulse, irregular heartbeat.

Protein

Protein is one of the most important nutrients we need to consume daily. Generally speaking, protein is not a problem for people with healthy kidneys because it is eliminated out of the body with the help of renal proteins and filtering units. But people with kidney disease need to be cautious about how much protein they consume because their body doesn't remove this nutrient properly.

Fluid

People with kidney disease need to manage fluid intake, especially in later stages. The reason leads us back to the main function of the kidneys, which is to balance the fluid levels and help expel the waste. Impaired function of the bean-shaped organs causes fluid buildup as they are unable to remove it properly. For example, dialysis patients have reduced the output of urine, so a higher intake of fluids can create unwanted and unnecessary pressure on the lungs and heart.

Chapter 3: Introduction to Renal Diet

Your mission, should you choose to accept it, is to ensure that you minimize waste buildup in your kidneys. To do that, you need to watch what you eat, carefully preparing or arranging your meals so that you receive the required nutrition, minus all the unnecessary components.

This is where a renal diet becomes an essential component of your life.

Before delving deeper into the diet itself, let us look at some of the important substances that people with CKD need to manage.

Sodium

If you have been enjoying your pasta, nachos, pizzas, juicy steaks, lip-smackin' burgers or practically any of your favorite savory food items, chances are that you have been consuming sodium. Why? Well, this mineral is commonly found in salt. Whether you use table salt or sea salt, you are going to find sodium in them.

If you have heard people claim that sodium is harmful to your body, then let me tell you that it is not entirely true. We need sodium in our body. The mineral helps our body maintain a balance in the levels of water within and around our cells. At the same time, it also maintains your blood pressure levels.

Surprised? You might have thought that sodium makes things worse, but there is a medical condition called hyponatremia, or "low blood sodium." When sodium levels drop to a low enough level, then you experience all the symptoms below:

- weakness
- nausea
- vomiting
- fatigue or low energy
- headache
- irritability

- muscle cramps or spasms
- confusion

In conclusion, sodium is essential for your body. But when you are on a renal diet, then you control the amount of salt that you add to your food. Since the kidneys are rather sensitive at this point, there is no need to exacerbate their condition by adding more sodium.

This might prove difficult for people since they are used to having salt as a flavoring ingredient in their foods. But that is why we are going to use recipes that are full of flavors that you will enjoy (more on that when we get started on the recipes).

Potassium

Potassium is one of those minerals that people might not think about too much as compared to calcium or sodium, but it nonetheless serves an important role in our body.

Apart from regulating fluids in the body, it also aids the body in passing messages between the body and the brain. Just like sodium, potassium is classified as an electrolyte, a term used to refer to a family of minerals that react in water. When potassium is dissolved in water, it produces positively charged ions. Using these ions, potassium can conduct electricity, which allows it to carry out some incredibly important functions. Take for example the messages that are communicated between the brain and the body. These messages are sent back and forth in the form of impulses. But one has to wonder; what exactly creates those impulses? It's not like our body has an inbuilt electrical generator.

The answer lies in the ions. We have already established that sodium and potassium are both electrolytes and produce ions. The impulses are created when sodium ions move into the cells and potassium ions move out of the cell. This movement changes the voltage of the cell, producing impulses. The way the impulses are created is similar to Morse code but takes place much faster (it has to for your body to react, manage processes, or perform tasks). When the level of potassium falls, the body's ability to generate nerve impulses gets affected.

Wait a minute. So potassium is good. Does that mean I am asking you to let your body give up on normal nerve impulses to keep your kidneys safe? Is that the only choice? That's a tough choice to make!

Relax. What we are going to do is avoid having too much potassium.

When the kidneys are not functioning properly, then the potassium buildup in the body could cause problems to the heart. More specifically, they could change the rhythm of the heartbeats, which could lead to a potential heart attack. But don't worry. This does not happen with just a mild increase in potassium. There has to be a significant increase to cause such a devastating result. Nevertheless, we are going to avoid even reaching a 'mild' increase. I placed the mild in quotes because there is no actual benchmark to gauge if the potassium content in your blood is mild or potentially life-threatening. It all depends on various factors in the body. I shall list down a few foods that are high in potassium that you should watch out for:

- Melons such as cantaloupe and honeydew (watermelon is acceptable)
- Oranges and orange juice
- Winter squash
- Pumpkin
- Bananas
- Prune juice
- Grapefruit juice
- Dried beans – all kinds

Try to also avoid granola bars (even though they are advertised as being nutritious) and bran cereals.

Phosphorus

Finally, we have phosphorus. This mineral makes up about 1% of your body weight. That may not seem like a lot in actuality, but remember that our body consists of a lot of water. For this reason, oxygen makes up 62% of our total body weight, followed by carbon at 18%, hydrogen at 9%, and nitrogen at 3%. But guess which are the next two major elements in the human body?

Calcium at 1.5%.

Phosphorus at 1%.

So you see, even though phosphorus makes up just 1% of the total body weight, it is still a significant element.

What is it used for?

Let me put it this way. Phosphorus is one of the reasons by you can smile wide. It is the reason your skin and other parts of the body are the way they are and do not just fall on the floor, like the way a piece of cloth might when you drop it. Phosphorus is responsible for the formation of your teeth and the bones that keep your body structure the way it currently is.

Pretty fantastic isn't it? We often nominate calcium as the main element in the formation of teeth and bones, but forget the less popular, and often overlooked, partner element that helps with the same task.

However, the fact that phosphorus keeps our teeth and bones healthy is something people eventually discover. What they don't discover is that phosphorus also plays an important role in helping the body use fats and carbohydrates. The mineral is truly important for the everyday function of the body.

When kidney problems strike us, we don't need the extra amount of phosphorus. While phosphorus is truly important for our bones and teeth, an excessive amount in the blood can lead to weaker bones. Since most of the food that we eat already includes phosphorus, we are going to try and avoid anything that has a high percentage of the mineral.

Fluids

Water sustains us. After all, 60% of the human adult's body is composed of water. This is why you might have heard of popular recommendations on how you should be having about eight glasses of water per day.

There is still a debate on exactly how much water is needed by an individual daily. But the fact remains; we need enough to avoid dehydration and keep the body functioning normally.

When you have kidney disease, you may not need as much fluid as you did before. The reason for this is that damaged kidneys do not dispose of extra fluids as well as they should. All the extra fluid in your body could be dangerous. It could cause swelling in various areas, high blood pressure, and heart problems. Fluid can also build up around your lungs, preventing you from breathing normally.

There is no measurement of how much fluid is considered as extra fluid. I strongly suggest that you should visit the doctor and get more information about fluid retention from him or her. The doctor will be able to guide you better and help you understand how much fluids you might require. The thing to understand here is that many of the foods that we eat, including fruits, vegetables, and most soups, have a water content in them as well. Getting to know your kidney's ability to hold on to fluids will aid you in preparing or planning better meals for yourself.

The Renal Diet

When we follow the renal diet, we are going to make use of all the information about various components and minerals of foods to prepare a meal that is as ideal for your body as possible. One of the renal diet's main aims is to manage the intake of sodium, potassium, and phosphorus. At the same time, the renal diet focuses on consuming high-quality protein and limiting the consumption of fluids. I believe that knowing about what you should eat and what you shouldn't go a long way in finding out if there is anything in particular that you should avoid (due to allergies for example).

So how exactly does the renal diet benefit you?

Preventing Diabetes and High Blood Pressure From Worsening

When you manage two of the biggest contributors of CKD, then you are delaying the effects of the disease greatly. You are getting out of a loop where either diabetes or high blood pressure makes the disease worse, further worsening either of the two conditions, which results in the disease entering a worse phase, and on it goes. This loop continues until it results in complete kidney failure.

Additionally, you might notice that your daily life becomes affected by CKD if you are not doing anything to manage the disease. You might find yourself losing focus on the things that you like, becoming less productive, and feeling too lethargic. You might also experience a greater degree of discomfort or exhaustion, even if you only have been walking at a normal pace.

A renal diet helps you avoid all the complications of diabetes and high blood pressure daily. Through careful planning, you might not feel as though your life has taken a heavy toll because of the disease. At the end of the day, you need to bring back as much normality in your life as possible and a renal diet helps you with that.

Prevents Cardiovascular Problems

Because a renal diet manages various aspects of our health, including the consumption of sodium, potassium, and phosphorus, it aids in preventing cardiovascular risk factors from developing (Cupisti, Aparicio & Barsotti, 2007). When you manage the sodium content in your body, you also ensure that the levels of cholesterol are low. When you have too much cholesterol in your blood, then it tends to accumulate in the walls of your arteries. This process is called atherosclerosis and is a type of heart disease.

Why is the accumulation of cholesterol in the heart harmful?

Let's take an example to highlight this point. Imagine a highway with six lanes. On a busy day, the lanes are usually filled. You notice that vehicles can get by without facing any congestion, but it does not mean that they have empty roads to use. The roads are good to drive on because there are no accidents or anything to halt the smooth flow of traffic. Now imagine that the government decides that they have to perform maintenance on four of the six lanes. They block these lanes and vehicles have to use two lanes for at least two miles. Imagine what would happen then. Think of the slow pace at which vehicles are going to move. In 2010, a reduction in road capacity caused a traffic jam in China that lasted for 12 days!

Now think of what happens when the same situation occurs in your body. Your arteries are the highways and the blood that has to flow to various parts of the body are the vehicles. Cholesterol is the problem that blocks lanes and restricts the movement of blood. When enough blood does not reach your heart, then you begin to suffer from a myriad of problems including chest pains and heart attacks.

Maintaining your cholesterol levels are important for healthy cardiovascular health. A renal diet ensures that you are avoiding foods that increase cholesterol.

Provides Essential Nutrients

The renal diet includes a lot of the good stuff and removes as much of the unnecessary stuff as possible. This means that the diet uses select ingredients to give you many vital nutrients in one meal. This ability of the diet to filter through various kinds of food to produce something extremely healthy for you is why it is popular among people with CKD who simply want to minimize the consumption of certain minerals.

Good Energy

One of the thoughts that zip through people's minds (I say 'zip' because it usually does not stay too long and you are going to find out why) is if they might receive the right about of energy from a renal diet. We are all used to consuming a certain type of food that includes numerous minerals and essential components. The renal diet is going to cut many of those components out of your diet. It's like looking at a five-story building, deciding that the top three stories don't matter and just deciding to bulldoze the unwanted floors! Indeed, a renal diet is going to feel like an extreme diet, since you are going to suddenly cut down on a lot of foods. You are going to 'bulldoze' them from your daily meals.

However, with the kind of food that you are going to eat, you won't have to worry about energy. When you are on a renal diet, you can perform many physical activities that you might have thought you won't be able to engage in after entering the diet.

You are going to get your energy from so many healthy and nutritious sources, as you will discover once you start reading through the recipes.

Five Tips for Slowing Down Kidney Disease

Having your kidneys function better for a longer period is one more day you don't have to worry about kidney failure. The more you slow down your CKD's progress, the fewer chances you have of finally looking for drastic kidney treatments. Some of the changes that you use for your kidneys also work to improve other organs in your body, such as your heart.

Just what are the tips that you need to follow to slow down kidney disease?

Tip #1: Maintain Your Blood Sugar in the Target Range

When you are checking blood sugar levels, you might find out that your blood sugar levels go through quite a few changes. It is not important to focus on these changes heavily when gauging the blood sugar levels, but they are important to know if you would like to get more details of your sugar levels. Before venturing further into understanding your glucose levels, I would like to first draw your attention to a particular measurement – mmol/L.

'Mmol' is short for millimole. A mole essentially calculates just how many atoms of a particular mineral or compound is present in a chemical process or reaction. A millimole is one-thousandth of a mole. The measurement is used to make precise calculations of the contents of fluids in our body, especially when it comes to blood sugar levels. The 'L' in mmol/L represent liters. What the measurement is trying to show you is the number of atoms of glucose or sugar (represented in mmol) is present in every liter of your blood. A typical adult will have anywhere between 4.7 to 5.5 liters of blood in their body. By using mmol/L, you get to know if you have high or low sugar content.

Tip #2: Exercise regularly

If you were already consuming foods that are healthy then it would also make sense if you were exercising regularly. Because regular physical activity will prevent weight gain and also regulate your blood pressure. But you should be careful about the amount of time you exercise or how much you exercise, especially if you aren't acclimatized to exercising. Don't overexert yourself if you are just getting started, because this would just increase the pressure on your kidneys and can also result in the breaking down of your muscles.

Tip #3: Be careful when making use of supplements

If you are consuming any supplements or any other herbal remedies, then you should be mindful of the amount you are consuming. Consuming excessive amount of vitamin supplements as well as any herbal extracts can prove to be harmful to the functioning of your kidneys. You should talk to your doctor before you start taking any supplements.

Tip #4: Quit smoking

Smoking causes damage to your blood vessels and this in turn would reduce the flow of blood to and in your kidneys. When the kidneys don't receive sufficient blood, they won't function like they are supposed to. Smoking also tends to increase your blood pressure and can also cause kidney cancer, apart from damaging your lungs.

Tip #5: Over-the-counter medication:

Whenever you are consuming any over-the-counter medications, then you shouldn't overdo it. Most of the common OTC medications tend to cause kidney damage if they are being consumed over a prolonged period of time. If your kidneys are healthy and if you consume these medicines for occasional minor ailments, then they don't pose a threat. But if you are taking them for any serious conditions like arthritis or chronic pain, then you should probably talk to your doctor before you start consuming them and you should also keep monitoring the functioning of your kidneys. If you know that you are a risk of renal failure, then you should keep getting regular screening of the functioning of your kidneys for making sure that they are functioning normally. If you have diabetes or high blood pressure, t is advisable that you get your kidneys screened for any dysfunction.

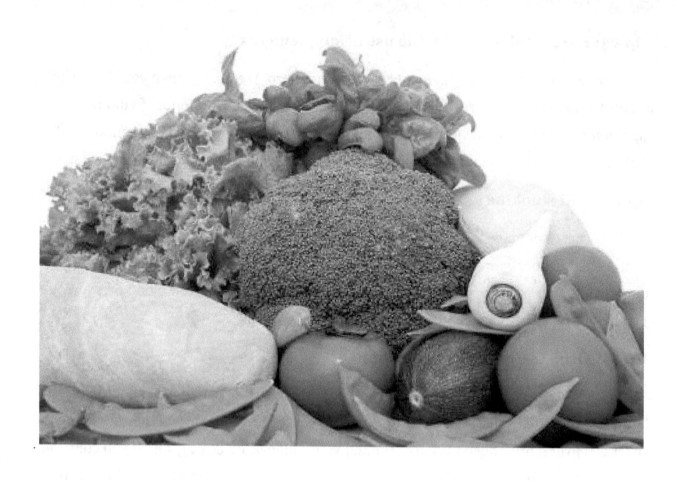

Chapter 4: Benefits of Renal Diet

The Renal diet controls your consumption of sodium, protein, potassium and phosphorous. A renal diet contributes to preventing renal failure. Below are a list of food/nutrients you should avoid preventing kidney-related problems:

Phosphate: Consumption of phosphate becomes dangerous when kidney failure reaches 80% and goes to the 4th/5th stage of kidney failure. So, it is better to lower your phosphate intake by counting the calories and minerals.

Protein: Being on a renal diet, you should intake 0.75 kg protein per day. Good source of protein are eggs, milk, cheese, meat, nuts, and fish.

Potassium: After getting diagnosed, if your results show your potassium level is high in the blood, then you should restrict your potassium intake. Baked and fried potatoes are very high in potassium. Leafy greens, fruit juices are high in potassium. You can still enjoy vegetables that are low in potassium.

Sodium: Adding salt is very important in our food, but when you are suffering from kidney problems, you have to omit or minimize your salt intake. Too much sodium intake can trigger high blood pressure and fluid retention in the body. You need to find substitutes that help season your food. Herbs and spices that are extracted from plants are a good option. Using garlic, pepper, mustard can increase the taste of your food without adding any salt. Avoid artificial "salts" that are low in sodium because they are high in potassium, which is also dangerous for kidney health.

Renal diets help people with kidney disease increase their quality of life.

Other types of food may be harmful to kidneys infected with a disease, so you need to make sure you have a sound knowledge of the infection and how it affects the body.

You don't want kidney disease, but there are ways to boost your well-being by changing your diet. In reality, renal diets help you manage your health and reduce kidney disease.

You need to remember—changing your diet won't heal everybody, but it can help everyone. This doesn't mean a diet is a cure-all, so don't think of this article as medical advice; it's more of a guide.

Your doctor can provide more guidance than this does and should always be informed or notified of any improvement in your condition.

If you have kidney problems, it's essential to regulate your health to help you feel better. There are entire books devoted to renal diets, or you can check with a registered dietitian for recommendations. Using a Kindle or iPad, you can even download and access these books instantly.

Dietitians have experience working with those with kidney problems and can give some general do's and don'ts to follow, such as control potassium intake—fruits like strawberries and apples are low in potassium, along with vegetables like cauliflower, cabbage and broccoli.

Track your phosphorous consumption—-creamers, pasta, cereals and rice are on the OK list.

Restrict liquid intake to 48 oz. This is the recommended level of fluid per day for renal diets— be sure to count fluid in items like grapes, ice cream, oranges, etc.

Track your salt intake—you'll need to be a tag reader to make sure you keep your salt intake low—-know what you're putting in your body and what it might contain.

Regulate your protein intake—maintain 5-7 ounces. Use egg replacements instead of normal eggs as a good technique for low protein consumption.

If you choose to use a dietitian, they can point you precisely to what you should and shouldn't consume, and why. Being aware of the effect food has on your body is important and can help you feel good every day. Also, this design is not an alternative to clinical guidelines. Yet renal diets help most kidney disease sufferers to become and stay healthier.

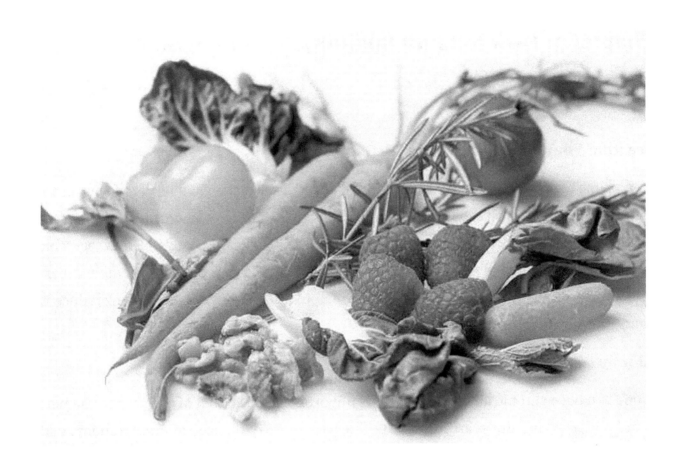

Chapter 5: How to Limit Sodium, Potassium And Phosphorus In The Diet

Treating Your Kidney Disease with Success

If you hope to successfully treat your chronic kidney disease, then you need to focus on your diet. This means that you should limit your protein, phosphorus, calcium, and sodium intake. Along with this, you should focus on eating a wide variety of healthy foods such as vegetables, fruits, and grains. Ideally, you should prioritize plant-based proteins over animal-based proteins, as the phosphorus in these is absorbed to a lesser degree, helping to reduce the dangerous phosphorus buildup in the bloodstream.

Kidney Disease Diet for Stages One Though Four

When you have chronic kidney disease, it is important to be careful of everything you put in your body, as your kidneys are less able to filter out waste or manage mineral contents in the bloodstream. Therefore, you want to eat in a way that reduces damage to your kidneys as much as possible. During the early stages of kidney disease, you will have more freedoms in what you eat, but as kidney disease progresses, you have to take more precautions.

Ideally, you want to consume a diet high in fruits and vegetables; with healthy fats and grains; some nuts, seeds, and beans; a small amount of protein and dairy; and low in sugar, sodium, phosphorus, magnesium, trans fats, and saturated fats.

Everyone needs protein in their diets. Even if you have chronic kidney disease and have to limit your protein intake, you still need some. This is because protein is used to fight infections, replace damaged cells, and maintain the mass of our muscles (including the heart). But how much protein should you be eating? There is not one standard number, as protein intake varies depending on a person's size, age, sex, and overall health.

There is a Recommended Dietary Allowance for healthy adults, which should be adjusted by a person's doctor if they have a condition such as chronic kidney disease. The recommendation is 0.8 grams of protein for every kilogram of body weight. This means that if an average healthy adult weighs 150, then they should be consuming 55 grams of protein daily to maintain their health requirements. If a person weighs 120 pounds, then they will need 44 grams of protein.

It is important to maintain adequate protein levels, as too little will cause muscle wasting, damage your heart, and result in increased infections. For most people, a slight increase in protein intake is not damaging, as their kidneys can filter out any waste byproducts and excrete them through the urine. However, this ability is diminished in people with chronic kidney disease. As these people have less kidney function, the waste byproducts are unable to be filtered out by the kidneys and result in a buildup of the waste in the bloodstream. This process increases the speed of kidney damage, worsening the disease at a rapid rate. Thankfully, studies have shown that if individuals with chronic kidney disease limit their protein intake, they can also slow the rate of progression of the disease and preserve kidney function.

A kidney specialist, known as a nephrologist, and a renal dietitian will be able to help a person determine how much protein they should consume when they have chronic kidney disease. They can calculate how much protein the body needs to maintain its normal function, while also reducing the protein intake to treat the disease and reduce kidney damage.

When eating protein, it is important to remember the difference between plant-based and animal-based proteins. While animal-based proteins contain all nine essential amino acids, making them a complete protein source, there are benefits to choosing plant-based protein sources instead. First, most sources of animal-based protein contain damaging saturated fats, which are generally not in plant-based proteins.

But, more importantly, phosphorus in plant-based proteins is less bioavailable than the phosphorus in animal-based proteins, which means your body will absorb less, thereby also lessening the damaging buildup of phosphorus in your bloodstream. When possible, choose plant-based protein sources over animal-based protein sources.

While animal-based sources are known as complete protein sources, there are some complete protein sources from plants. These mainly include soy products such as tofu, beans paired with rice, buckwheat, quinoa, and chia seeds. You can also find protein in many vegetables, grains, nuts, seeds, beans, and lentils. These are also high in fiber, which helps to lower blood sugar and cholesterol!

When you do choose animal-based protein sources, the best options that are low in saturated fat are fish, white meat poultry, and low-fat dairy products.

Let's have a look at some ways you can get a daily dose of protein. For this example, the protein requirement will be 50-60 grams, but you will need to discuss your specific protein needs with your doctor.

- Quinoa, cooked - 5 cup
- Yogurt, low-fat - 5 cup
- Beans, cooked - 5 cup
- Chicken breast – 4 ounces

With this example, a person can consume 53 grams of protein over their day. It also contains 707 milligrams of phosphorus, 176 milligrams of sodium, 320 milligrams of calcium, and 1090 milligrams of potassium.

Limit the Sodium, Phosphorus, Potassium, and Calcium:

Sodium is found in many foods; it is more than only table salt. It is important to be careful with this mineral and your consumption of it, especially when you have high blood pressure or chronic kidney disease. This is because sodium affects the water balance in your body and can greatly raise your blood pressure, in the process causing more kidney damage and increasing your risk of heart disease. Thankfully, your doctor can run a simple blood test to see the mineral levels in your bloodstream, which will allow you to know whether or not your sodium levels are too high.

If your blood pressure is at a healthy level, and you are only in the early stages of chronic kidney disease, you can aim for two to three grams of sodium a day. However, if you are in the later stages of kidney disease with high blood pressure, you should reduce your sodium consumption to be below two grams daily.

To cut your sodium consumption, you should avoid:

- Table salt
- Sea salt
- Garlic salt
- Seasoning salt
- Soy sauce
- Onion salt
- Celery salt
- Meat tenderizer
- Lemon pepper.
- Oyster sauce
- Teriyaki sauce
- Barbecue sauce
- Cured foods, such as meats and vegetables
- Lunch meats

Most fast foods and highly processed foods are high in sodium, meaning that cooking at home is your best option. This doesn't mean you have to cook difficult and elaborate meals; they can be simple and easy. Since you cannot include salt, instead enjoy a wide selection of sodium-free spices and herbs. Whenever you cook with canned foods, you should drain off the liquid and then rinse the food in warm water, to remove excess sodium. Lastly, always read ingredient labels to check the sodium content.

It is important to watch your phosphorus levels, to prevent a buildup in your bloodstream. Ask your doctor how much phosphorus you should aim for as your daily intake. In general, when a person develops late-stage kidney disease, their doctor will advise them to consume no more than one gram of phosphorus daily.

You can limit your phosphorus intake by limiting dairy consumption, cutting back on meats and fish, reading ingredient and nutrition labels to avoid high phosphorus ingredients, avoiding dark-colored sodas, increasing fresh fruits and vegetables, and consuming more rice and corn products.

Your doctor will likely recommend that you reduce your calcium intake, which shouldn't be difficult as foods high in calcium are generally also high in phosphorus. This means you naturally will not be consuming much calcium. The easiest way to reduce your calcium intake is to limit dairy products, bone-in fish, seeds, and fortified foods.

Lastly, you should limit your potassium intake. This mineral is really important, but most people consume much more than they need. While this is not generally a problem, it becomes one for people with decreased renal function as their kidneys are no longer able to filter out the excess potassium, causing a buildup in the bloodstream. This can be more difficult to avoid, as many foods are rich in potassium, such as fruits and vegetables. In general, you don't want to consume any more than two grams of potassium daily.

Try to limit potassium-rich foods, such as:

- Tomatoes
- Potatoes
- Sweet Potatoes
- Cranberries
- Blueberries
- Strawberries
- Raspberries
- Plums
- Star fruit
- Avocados
- Bananas
- Whole-wheat bread
- Brown rice

- Dairy

- Oranges

- Apricots

- Winter Squash

- Beets

- Dark leafy greens

- Dried fruits

- Parsnips

- Rutabaga

Kidney Disease Diet for Stage Five and Dialysis Patients

When you are in the fifth stage of chronic kidney disease, in which your kidneys fail and you most likely begin dialysis, you have to take even more precautions than you do in stages one through four of kidney disease. This means that you have to be even more careful in which foods you eat, how much protein you consume, and the number of minerals in your meals.

Since you will now be on dialysis, you will need to limit your fluid intake and foods that cause a buildup of waste or excess minerals int eh bloodstream. Your doctor, renal dietitian, and the dialysis center should be able to help you monitor your diet and answer any questions you might need. These doctors, dietitians, and nurses are there to help and can help you customize your diet to ideally fit your needs.

If you also have high blood pressure, high cholesterol, or diabetes, you will be happy to know that this diet will not only benefit your chronic kidney disease but your other conditions, as well.

In general, dialysis patients need to:

- Consume more protein-rich foods

- Consume less sodium, phosphorus, and potassium

- Control fluid intake including water, tea, coffee, juices, and other beverages

Fluids:

While many people in today's day and age do not drink enough water, the same is not true of dialysis patients. People who are undergoing dialysis therapy can easily consume too much water, causing a fluid overload known as hypervolemia. The kidneys are responsible for balancing the amount of fluid in your body, but when this is disrupted is can negatively affect your health, causing swelling and difficulty breathing.

When a person begins dialysis treatment, their kidneys are no longer able to balance the amount of fluid is in their body. This results in them being unable to remove enough fluid, causing a buildup in the body. This is also why you have to be even more vigilant in reducing sodium intake, as sodium affects your body's fluid levels. Thankfully, if you can carefully manage both your fluid and sodium intake, your dialysis treatments should be able to maintain the correct amount of these two in your body, removing any excess.

If you are worried you may have consumed too much liquid you should watch for symptoms of swelling in your hands, feet, and face; shortness of breath; high blood pressure; cramping, headaches, and bloating; and heart problems such as changes in your heart rate or palpitations.

You can better manage your fluid intake by tracking how much you are drinking. Some people may prefer to do this with a small notebook they can keep on them, although it is generally easier to use a smartphone app. There are many apps designed to track your liquid intake. Remember, when tracking your intake don't only track water, but all the liquid you consume.

You can better manage your thirst by sucking on sugar-free hard candies, frozen grapes, and ice chips. These can help you to avoid drinking too much between your dialysis therapy sessions.

Keep in mind that sodium causes your body to hold onto water. You will have to be even more careful with your sodium intake than you were in earlier stages of kidney disease.

Follow the fluid recommendations given to you by your doctor and dialysis team. This will vary from person to person based on their body and various lifestyle factors. However, most people are instructed to limit their fluid intake to only thirty-two ounces daily.

If you have concerns about developing fluid overload, then talk with your healthcare team. They may need to adjust your dialysis treatments to account for any concerns, such as including either longer or more frequent dialysis treatments.

Meat and Protein:

While people in earlier stages of kidney disease need to limit their protein intake, patients in stage five who are on dialysis will be required to increase their protein intake. By increasing your protein, you can maintain healthy blood protein levels and improve your overall health.

Try choosing fish, poultry, and eggs while generally avoiding red meat, which is high in saturated fats. In general, you will want to eat eight to ten ounces of high-protein ingredients, such as meat, dairy.

Beans, lentils, peas, nuts, seeds, and peanuts will have to be eaten in moderation. Keep in mind that these foods are high in phosphorus and potassium, so you should only eat small servings of them when it does not cause you to go over your daily limit.

Grains and Cereals:

Grains and cereals can be a great option, in some cases. Not everyone can enjoy these foods as if you are having trouble managing your blood sugar; they could spike it even more. Therefore, it is generally best for diabetic patients to limit grains.

When choosing grains try to avoid whole-grain or high-fibre varieties, such as brown rice and whole-wheat bread. While these are generally better options for healthy people, the same is not true for those with chronic kidney disease, as they contain a larger amount of phosphorus. Instead, choose the processed forms of grains such as white rice, pasta, and white bread.

Fruits and Vegetables:

When consuming fruits and vegetables, you want to select varieties that are low in phosphorus and potassium. It is helpful that canned fruits are lower in potassium than the fresh alternates. On the other hand, canned vegetables have more sodium and should be rinsed off before using.

It is a good idea to download a diet app on your smartphone and track what you eat. Try to find an app option that will give you the full nutritional details of what you are eating, so that you can easily track your mineral intake and reduce the risk of overconsumption.

Try to consume two or three servings of low-potassium fruits daily, such as:

- Apple – 1
- Pear –.5
- Peach – 1
- Tangerine – 1
- Plums – 2
- Cherries – 10
- Berries - .5 cup
- Fruit cocktail, drained - .5 cup
- Grapes – 15
- Pineapple, canned, drained - .5 cup
- Watermelon, small wedge – 1

Consume two to three servings of low-potassium vegetables daily. Keep in mind that they will all have some potassium, which you need to track so that you aren't consuming more than you believe.

Some options include:

- Cabbage
- Radishes

- Broccoli
- String Beans
- Lettuce
- Eggplant
- Celery
- Watercress
- Peppers
- Cauliflower
- Carrots
- Eggplant
- Yellow Squash
- Zucchini
- Onions

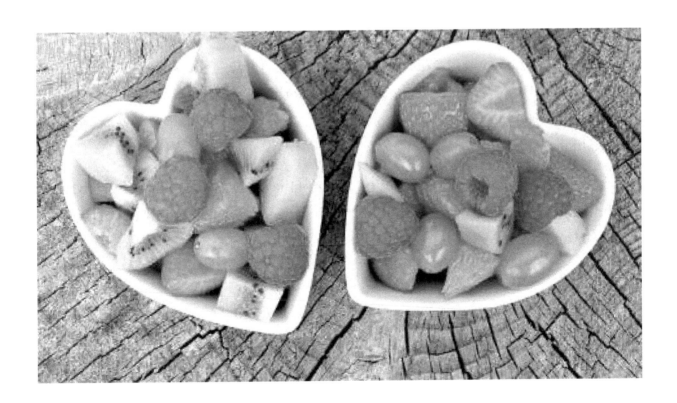

Chapter 6: What You Can Eat and What You Can Avoid in Renal Diet

Food to Eat

The renal diet aims to cut down the amount of waste in the blood. When people have kidney dysfunction, the kidneys are unable to remove and filter waste properly. When waste is left in the blood, it can affect the electrolyte levels of the patient. With a kidney diet, kidney function is promoted, and the progression of complete kidney failure is slowed down.

The renal diet follows a low intake of protein, phosphorus, and sodium. It is necessary to consume high-quality protein and limit some fluids. For some people, it is important to limit calcium and potassium.

Promoting a renal diet, here are the substances which are critical to be monitored:

Sodium and its role in the body

Most natural foods contain sodium. Some people think that sodium and salt are interchangeable. However, salt is a compound of chloride and sodium. There might be either salt or sodium in other forms in the food we eat. Due to the added salt, processed foods include a higher level of sodium.

Apart from potassium and chloride, sodium is one of the most crucial body's electrolytes. The main function of electrolytes is controlling the fluids when they are going out and in of the body's cells and tissues.

With sodium:

- Blood volume and pressure are regulated
- Muscle contraction and nerve function are regulated
- Acid-based balance of the blood is regulated
- The amount of fluid the body eliminates and keeps is balanced

Why is it important to monitor sodium intake for people with kidney issues?

Since the kidneys of kidney disease patients are unable to reduce excess fluid and sodium from the body adequately, too much sodium might be harmful. As fluid and sodium build up in the bloodstream and tissues, they might cause:

- Edema: swelling in face, hands, and legs
- Increased thirst
- High blood pressure
- Shortness of breath
- Heart failure

The ways to monitor sodium intake:

- Avoid processed foods
- Be attentive to serving sizes
- Read food labels
- Utilize fresh meats instead of processed
- Choose fresh fruits and veggies
- Compare brands, choosing the ones with the lowest sodium levels
- Utilize spices that do not include salt
- Ensure the sodium content is less than 400 mg per meal and not more than 150 mg per snack
- Cook at home, not adding salt
- Foods to eat with lower sodium content:
- Fresh meats, dairy products, frozen veggies, and fruits
- Fresh herbs and seasonings like rosemary, oregano, dill, lime, cilantro, onion, lemon, and garlic
- Corn tortilla chips, pretzels, no salt added crackers, unsalted popcorn

Potassium and its role in the body

The main function of potassium is keeping muscles working correctly and the heartbeat regular. This mineral is responsible for maintaining electrolyte and fluid balance in the bloodstream. The kidneys regulate the proper amount of potassium in the body, expelling excess amounts in the urine.

Monitoring potassium intake

- Limit high potassium food
- Select only fresh fruits and veggies
- Limit dairy products and milk to 8 oz per day
- Avoid potassium chloride
- Read labels on packaged foods
- Avoid seasonings and salt substitutes with potassium

Foods to eat with lower potassium:

- Fruits: watermelon, tangerines, pineapple, plums, peaches, pears, papayas, mangoes, lemons and limes, honeydew, grapefruit/grapefruit juice, grapes/grape juice, clementine/satsuma, cranberry juice, berries, and apples/applesauce, apple juice
- Veggies: summer squash (cooked), okra, mushrooms (fresh), lettuce, kale, green beans, eggplant, cucumber, corn, onions (raw), celery, cauliflower, carrots, cabbage, broccoli (fresh), bamboo shoots (canned), and bell peppers
- Plain Turkish delights, marshmallows and jellies, boiled fruit sweets, and peppermints
- Shortbread, ginger nut biscuits, plain digestives
- Plain flapjacks and cereal bars
- Plain sponge cakes like Madeira cake, lemon sponge, jam sponge
- Corn-based and wheat crisps
- Whole grain crispbreads and crackers

- Protein and other foods (bread (not whole grain), pasta, noodles, rice, eggs, canned tuna, turkey (white meat), and chicken (white meat)

Phosphorus and its role in the body

This mineral is essential in bone development and maintenance. Phosphorus helps in the development of connective organs and tissue and assists in muscle movement. Extra phosphorus is possible to be removed by healthy kidneys. However, it is impossible with kidney dysfunction. High levels of phosphorus make bones weak by pulling calcium out of your bones. It might lead to dangerous calcium deposits in the heart, eyes, lungs, and blood vessels.

Monitoring phosphorus intake

- Pay attention to serving size
- Eat fresh fruits and veggies
- Eat smaller portions of foods that are rich in protein
- Avoid packaged foods
- Keep a food journal

Foods to eat with low phosphorus level:

- grapes, apples
- lettuce, leeks
- Carbohydrates (white rice, corn and rice Cereal, popcorn, pasta, crackers (not wheat), white bread)
- Meat (sausage, fresh meat)

Protein

Damaged kidneys are unable to remove protein waste, so they accumulate in the blood. The amount of protein to consume differs depending on the stage of CKD. Protein is critical for tissue maintenance, and it is necessary to eat the proper amount of it according to the particular stage of kidneys disease.

Sources of protein for vegetarians:

- Vegans (allowing only plant-based foods): Wheat protein and whole grains, nut butter, soy protein, yogurt or soy milk, cooked no salt added canned and dried beans and peas, unsalted nuts.
- Lacto vegetarians (allowing dairy products, milk, and plant-based foods): reduced-sodium or low-sodium cottage cheese.
- Lacto-ovo vegetarians (allowing eggs, dairy products, milk, and plant-based foods): eggs.

Food to Avoid

Food with high sodium content:

- Onion salt, marinades, garlic salt, teriyaki sauce, and table salt
- Pepperoni, bacon, ham, lunch meat, hot dogs, sausage, processed meats
- Ramen noodles, canned produce, and canned soups
- Marinara sauce, gravy, salad dressings, soy sauce, BBQ sauce, and ketchup
- Chex Mix, salted nuts, Cheetos, crackers, and potato chips
- Fast food

Food with a high potassium level:

- Fruits: dried fruit, oranges/orange juice, prunes/prune juice, kiwi, nectarines, dates, cantaloupe, bananas, black currants, damsons, cherries, grapes, and apricots.
- Vegetables: tomatoes/tomato sauce/tomato juice, sweet potatoes, beans, lentils, split peas, spinach (cooked), pumpkin, potatoes, mushrooms (cooked), chile peppers, chard, Brussels sprouts (cooked), broccoli (cooked), baked beans, avocado, butternut squash, and acorn squash.
- Protein and other foods: peanut butter, molasses, granola, chocolate, bran, sardines, fish, bacon, ham, nuts and seeds, yogurt, milkshakes, and milk.
- Coconut-based snacks, nut-based snacks, fudge, and toffee.

- Cakes containing marzipan.
- Potato crisps.

Foods with high phosphorus:

- Dairy products: pudding, ice cream, yogurt, cottage cheese, cheese, and milk.
- Nuts and seeds: sunflower seeds, pumpkin seeds, pecans, peanut butter, pistachios, cashews, and almonds.
- Dried beans and peas: soybeans, split peas, refried beans, pinto beans, lentils, kidney beans, garbanzo beans, black beans, and baked beans.
- Meat: veal, turkey, liver, lamb, beef, bacon, fish, and seafood.
- Carbohydrates: whole grain products, oatmeal, and bran cereals.

Renal Diet Shopping List

Vegetables:

- Arugula (raw)
- Alfalfa sprouts
- Bamboo shoots
- Asparagus
- Beans - pinto, wax, fava, green
- Bean sprouts
- Bitter melon (balsam pear)
- Beet greens (raw)
- Broccoli
- Broad beans (boiled, fresh)
- Cactus
- Cabbage - red, swamp, Napa/ Suey Choy, skunk
- Carrots
- Calabash
- Celery

- Cauliflower
- Chayote
- Celeriac (cooked)
- Collard greens
- Chicory
- Cucumber
- Corn
- Okra
- Onions
- Pepitas
- (Green) Peas
- Peppers
- Radish
- Radicchio
- Seaweed
- Rapini (raw)
- Shallots
- Spinach (raw)
- Snow peas
- Dandelion greens (raw)
- Daikon
- Plant Leaves
- Drumstick
- Endive
- Eggplant
- Fennel bulb
- Escarole
- Fiddlehead greens

- Ferns
- Hearts of Palm
- GaiLan
- Irishmoss
- Hominy
- Jicama,raw
- Jew'sEar
- Leeks
- Kale(raw)
- Mushrooms (rawwhite)
- Lettuce (raw)
- Nopales
- Mustardgreens
- Swisschard (raw)
- Squash
- Turnip
- Tomatillos (raw)
- Watercress
- Turnip greens
- Wax beans
- Water chestnuts (canned)
- Winter melon
- Wax gourd
- Zucchini (raw)

Fruits:

- Acerola Cherries
- Apple
- Blackberries

- Asian Pear
- Boysenberries
- Blueberries
- Cherries
- Casaba melon
- Clementine
- Chokeberries
- Crabapples
- Cloudberries
- Feijoa
- Cranberries (fresh)
- Grapefruit
- Gooseberries
- Pomegranate
- Grapes
- Rambutan
- Quince
- Rhubarb
- Raspberries (fresh or frozen)
- Jujubes
- Golden Berry
- Kumquat
- Jackfruit
- Lingonberries
- Lemon
- Loganberries
- Lime
- Lychees

- Longans
- Mango
- Mandarin orange
- Peach
- Mangosteen
- Pineapple
- Pear
- Plum
- Pitanga
- Strawberries
- Rose-apple
- Tangerine
- Tangelo
- Watermelon

Bread products:

Packaged bread:

- Dimpflmeier Holzofen Art Brot-Real Stone Bread
- Country Harvest Vitality White with Whole Wheat
- Stonemill Sourdough Classic French
- Dimpflmeier Viking French Stick Bread
- Wonder White Thin Sandwich
- Wonder White + Fibre Bread
- Naan Bread
- Chapati/Roti
- Pita Bread
- Dempster's Smart White with 16 Whole Grains
- Wonder White with Fibre English Muffin

- Silver Hills Bakery Little Big, Steady Eddie

Packaged Bagels:

- Dempster's Original Bagels
- Stonemill Swiss Muesli Bagels

Hamburger/Hot Dog Buns:

- Wonder White Hamburger Bun
- Wonder White Hot Dog buns
- Dempster's Hot Dog Bun

Tortillas and Taco Shells:

- Old El Paso Flour Tortillas
- White flour or corn-based tortillas
- Old El Paso Taco Shells

Fresh Meat, Seafood, and Poultry:

- Chicken
- Beef and Ground Beef
- Goat
- Duck
- Wild Game
- Pork
- Lamb
- Veal
- Turkey
- Fish

Milk, Eggs, and Dairy:

Milk:

- Milk (½-1 cup/day)

Non-Dairy Milk:

- Almond Fresh (Original, Unsweetened, Vanilla)
- Almond Breeze (Original, Vanilla, Vanilla Unsweetened, Original Unsweetened)
- Silk True Almond Beverage (Unsweetened Original, Original, Vanilla, Unsweetened Vanilla)
- Good Karma Flax Delight (Vanilla, Original, Unsweetened)
- Rice Dream Rice Drink (Vanilla Classic, Non-Enriched Original Classic)
- Silk Soy Beverage (Original, Vanilla, Unsweetened)
- Natura Organic Fortified Rice Beverage (Original, Vanilla)
- PC Organics Fortified Rice Beverage

Coffee Creamer:

- Nestle Coffee-Mate (Original Fat-Free, Original, Original Low Fat)

Cheese:

- Feta
- Brie
- Goat Cheese, Soft
- Grated Parmesan Cheese
- Nanak Paneer President's Choice Bocconcini
- Liberte Fresh Cheese, Crème Fraiche
- Western Pressed Dry Cottage Cheese 0.1% or 0.5%, No Salt
- Trestelle Bocconcini, 40% Light Bocconcini, Mascarpone
- Lucerne Cottage Cheese, 2% No-Added-Salt

Other Dairy Products:

- Non-Hydrogenated Margarine (Salt-Free or Regular)
- Butter (Unsalted or Regular)
- Whipping Cream
- Sour Cream
- Whipped Cream

Eggs:

- Egg Beaters
- Fresh eggs, all types

Tofu:

- Tofu (soft)

Salt-Free Seasonings:

- McCormack Salt-Free Garlic and Herb, All-Purpose
- Clubhouse La Grille No Salt Added Chicken Seasoning, No Salt Added Steak Spice
- Allspice
- Anise
- Mrs. Dash
- Caraway seeds
- Celery seeds
- Cardamom
- Basil
- Bay Leaves
- Coriander
- Curry powder
- Cumin

- Chives
- Cinnamon
- Cloves
- Cilantro
- Garlic powder
- Ginger
- Dill
- Fennel
- Fenugreek
- Nutmeg
- Mace
- Mustard
- Marjoram
- Paprika
- Pepper (Black or Cayenne)
- Parsley
- Onion powder/flakes
- Oregano
- Rosemary
- Poultry seasoning
- Poppy seeds
- Tarragon
- Turmeric
- Thyme
- Saffron
- Savory
- Sage

List of Juices and Drinks for Renal Diet:

- Sparkling water
- Water
- Tea (Regular, Decaffeinated, or Herbal)
- Coffee (Decaffeinated or Regular)
- Club Soda
- Crystal Light flavor crystals
- Ginger Ale, Green Tea Ginger Ale, Diet Ginger Ale
- Cream Soda
- Pineapple juice
- Orange Pop
- Grape Pop
- Root Beer
- Sprite or Diet Sprite
- 7-Up or Diet 7-Up
- Apple Juice
- Tonic Water
- Apricot nectar
- Apple Cider
- Cranberry cocktail
- Cranberry Juice
- Grape juice
- Five Alive
- Peach nectar
- Lemonade
- Pear nectar

Dishes the Dialysis Patient Can Order at Restaurants

Breakfast

Poor Choices - Better Choices

☐ Salted cured meats or fish like ham, lox, sausage, and Canadian bacon - ☐ Eggs

☐ Omelets above meats or with cheese, breakfast burritos, fast-food breakfast sandwiches - ☐ Omelets with low-potassium vegetables like squash or mushrooms

☐ Bran muffins and biscuits - ☐ Toast, English muffins, bagels, croissants, blueberry, or plain muffins

☐ Hash brown potatoes - ☐ Pancakes, French toast, waffles

☐ Gravy or real maple syrup - ☐ Margarine, jelly, cinnamon, honey, sugar, imitation syrup, and pancake

☐ Fruits and juices like a fresh grapefruit half or orange juice - ☐ Low-potassium fruits and juices like apple juice or applesauce

☐ Granola with nuts and bran cereals, seeds or wheat germ - ☐ Cold and hot cereals

☐ Pastries containing chocolate, coconut, nuts, or caramel - ☐ Sweet rolls, fruit pastry, coffee cake

Beverages

Poor Choices - Better Choices

☐ Cocktails mixed with tomato juice, fruit juice, milk, cream, vegetable cocktail, or ice cream - ☐ Cocktails mixed with ginger ale, club soda, soft drinks (except colas), or tonic water

☐ Beer - ☐ Wine, white, or red when potassium is counted.

☐ Dark cola - ☐ Non-cola soft drinks like 7UP, Sprite, or orange soda

☐ Cocoa, milkshakes, milk, cocoa mixes - ☐ Iced coffee or tea

☐ Orange juice-type drinks, vegetable juice, tomato juice - ☐ Limeade, lemonade, water

Salads

Poor Choices - Better Choices

☐ Spinach, tomato, artichoke, avocado, kidney beans, seeds, garbanzo beans, nuts - ☐ Lettuce, cabbage, cauliflower, beets, celery, jicama, cucumber, onions, green peas, beans, radishes, sweet peppers, sprouts

☐ Potato salad - ☐ Coleslaw

☐ Three-bean salad - ☐ Beet salad

☐ Greek salad with relishes, olives, pickles - ☐ Macaroni salad, pasta salad

☐ Salad containing melon, bananas, oranges, kiwi, or dried fruit - ☐ Canned peaches or pears, canned fruit cocktail, mandarin oranges, fresh or canned pineapple.

Appetizers

Poor Choices - Better Choices

☐ Cheese fondue, cottage cheese, other cheese dishes, and anchovies - ☐ Caesar salad with shrimp or chicken

☐ Cheese sticks, quiche - ☐ Chicken, steak or pork tostadas

☐ Oysters - ☐ Crab cakes, fried calamari, steamed clams, most shrimp dishes

☐ Potato skins, nachos - ☐ Crab Louis salad

☐ Chopped liver or pâté; smoked or salted meat, poultry or fish like ham, smoked turkey or lox; soup, consomme or bouillon - ☐ Green salad with fish or meat, or chef's salad without cheese or ham

Entrées

Poor Choices - Better Choices

☐ Lamb or beef stew, onions and liver, salted or cured meats (ham, sausage, corned beef, prosciutto, chorizo) - ☐ Beef (grilled or broiled steaks, burgers with no cheese, hot roast or prime rib roast beef sandwiches), chicken (fried, baked, roasted or grilled), leg of lamb, veal, lamb chops, meatloaf

☐ Bouillabaisse, lobster Newburg, oysters, lox - ☐ Seafood (steamed, grilled, or poached), or fish

☐ Sauces (especially tomato or cheese), gravies - ☐ Meat kabobs or seafood

☐ Bean dishes, chili con carne, chili beans - ☐ Fajitas, chicken, or meat tacos (no tomatoes or cheese)

☐ Omelets with bacon, ham, cheese, sausage - ☐ Omelets with allowed vegetables and sauce which is served on the side

☐ Submarine sandwiches, BLT, toasted cheese, Reuben, bacon hamburger, tuna (canned) salad - ☐ Sandwiches (no cheese): chicken, roast beef, egg, turkey, fresh seafood sandwich, hot roast beef, or turkey

Side dishes

Poor Choices - Better Choices

☐ Pasta in tomato sauce - ☐ Noodles or pasta, macaroni salad, pesto pasta

☐ Yams, fried rice, sweet potatoes, white potatoes - ☐ Steamed rice, rice with peas, rice pilaf

☐ Barbecued or baked beans, refried beans - ☐ Unsalted breadsticks, rolls, or bread

☐ Higher-potassium vegetables, such as tomatoes, collard greens, spinach, acorn squash, artichokes, and others - ☐ Lower-potassium vegetables, such as asparagus, cooked carrots, cabbage, eggplant, corn, green peas, corn on the cob, zucchini, coleslaw, and lettuce salad

Desserts

Poor Choices - Better Choices

☐ Cakes rich in coconut, chocolate, nuts, or dried fruit, like carrot, chocolate mousse, fruit, or German chocolate cake - ☐ Lemon, apple, spice, pound, a yellow, or white cake might be topped with low potassium fruit and whipped cream

☐ Brownies, coconut macaroons, chocolate, snickerdoodles - ☐ Sugar cookies, lemon cream, vanilla wafers, and butter cookies

☐ Frozen yogurt or ice cream - ☐ Fruit ice, sorbet, sherbet

☐ Fruits higher in potassium, such as oranges, bananas or kiwi - ☐ Lower-potassium fruit desserts, such as strawberry shortcake, berries, gelatin desserts

☐ Pies, such as chocolate cream, coconut, banana cream, minced meat, pumpkin, pecan, sweet potato, or cheesecake - ☐ Pies, cobblers, or tarts made with blueberry, apple, cherry, strawberry, or lemon meringue

Fast food

Poor Choices - Better Choices

☐ Large hamburgers or cheeseburgers - ☐ Junior-size or regular hamburgers.

☐ Sandwiches with bacon, cheese, or sauces - ☐ Turkey sandwiches or roast beef

☐ Breaded, or fried chicken sandwiches, chicken strips, or nuggets - ☐ Broiled or grilled chicken sandwiches, chicken salad, or tuna

☐ French fries, baked potato, potato chips, baked beans, potato salad - ☐ Unsalted onion rings

☐ Pickles, or high-potassium foods from the salad bar; limiting tomatoes - ☐ Lettuce salads, macaroni salad, coleslaw

☐ Cola sodas and milkshakes - ☐ Non-cola soda, milkshakes, lemonade, and cola sodas tea, water, and coffee

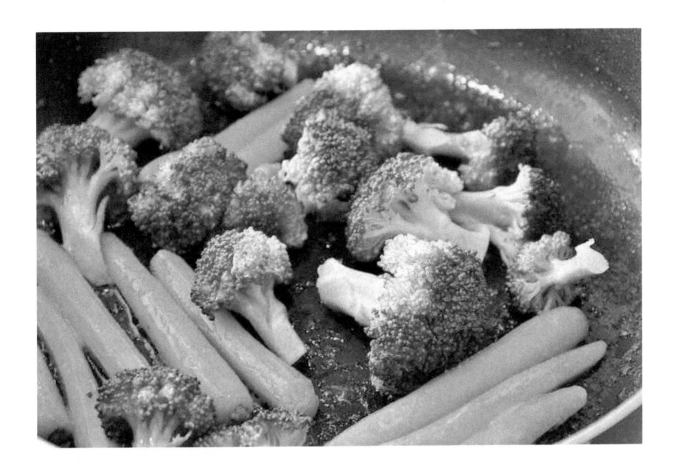

Chapter 7: Top 10 Foods to Eat for Kidney Health

There is a distinct connection between the health and function of our kidneys and the way we eat. How we eat and the foods we choose make a significant impact on how well we feel and our overall well-being. Making changes to your diet is often necessary to guard against medical conditions, and while eating well can treat existing conditions, healthy food choices can also help prevent many other conditions from developing – including kidney disease.

When we make changes to our diet, we often focus on the restrictions or foods we should avoid. While this is important, it's also vital to learn about the foods and nutrients we need to maintain good health and prevent disease. Consider the related conditions that contribute to high blood pressure and type 2 diabetes, and the dietary changes often suggested to treat and, in some successful cases, reverse the damage of these conditions. Dietary changes for the treatment and prevention of disease often focus on limiting salt, sugar, and trans fats from our food choices, while increasing minerals, protein, and fiber, among other beneficial nutrients. The renal diet also focuses on eliminating, or at least limiting, the consumption of various ingredients to aid our kidneys to function better and to prevent further damage from occurring.

The Best Foods on a Renal Diet

Many foods work well within the renal diet, and once you see the available variety, it will not seem as restrictive or difficult to follow. The key is focusing on the foods with a high level of nutrients, which make it easier for the kidneys to process waste by not adding too much that the body needs to discard. Balance is a major factor in maintaining and improving long-term renal function.

Egg Whites

Eggs are high in protein and eating them in excess can put a lot of pressure on kidneys that are not functioning at their peak. There is the option of limiting the number of eggs consumed to two per day, or using just the egg whites instead, as they provide the required nutrients without over-taxing the kidneys. Egg whites can be used in a variety of dishes just like whole eggs, such as omelets, scrambled eggs, soups, and stir fry dishes. For people on dialysis, this is a healthier and safer option than using the full egg.

Garlic

Excellent, vitamin-rich food for the immune system, garlic is a tasty substitute for salt in a variety of dishes. It acts as a significant source of vitamin C and B6 while aiding the kidneys in ridding the body of unwanted toxins. It's a great, healthy way to add flavor for skillet meals, pasta, soups, and stews.

Berries

All berries are considered a good renal diet food due to their high level of fiber, antioxidants, and delicious taste, making them an easy option to include as a light snack or as an ingredient in smoothies, salads, and light desserts. Just one handful of blueberries can provide almost one day's vitamin C requirement, as well as a boost of fiber, which is good for weight loss and maintenance.

Cabbage

For renal health, consider cabbage a superfood! Not only is this vegetable low in phosphorus, sodium, and potassium, it's an excellent source of minerals and vitamins that provide many of the required nutrients needed for a healthy, balanced diet. It's a good support for the digestive system and weight management, in addition to helping the kidneys. Cabbage is also a versatile food that can be used in a variety of dishes and cuisines, such as curries, baked cabbage rolls, soups, skillet meals, and salads. All varieties of cabbage are excellent, from savoy to red cabbage, and just a moderate portion is all that's needed to enjoy its nutritional benefits.

Bell Peppers

Flavorful and easy to enjoy both raw and cooked, bell peppers offer a good source of vitamin C, vitamin A, and fiber. Along with other kidney-friendly foods, they make the detoxification process much easier while boosting your body's nutrient level to prevent further health conditions and reduce existing deficiencies.

Onions

This nutritious and tasty vegetable is excellent as a companion to garlic in many dishes, or on its own. Like garlic, onions can provide flavor as an alternative to salt, and provides a good source of vitamin C, vitamin B, manganese, and fiber, as well. Adding just one quarter or half of the onion is often enough for most meals, because of its strong, pungent flavor.

Macadamia Nuts

If you enjoy nuts and seeds as snacks, you may soon learn that many contain high amounts of phosphorus and should be avoided or limited as much as possible. Fortunately, macadamia nuts are an easier option to digest and process, as they contain much lower amounts of phosphorus and make an excellent substitute for other nuts. They are a good source of other nutrients, as well, such as vitamin B, copper, manganese, iron, and healthy fats.

Pineapple

Unlike other fruits that are high in potassium, pineapple is an option that can be enjoyed more often than bananas and kiwis. Citrus fruits are generally high in potassium as well, so if you find yourself craving an orange or grapefruit, choose pineapple instead. In addition to providing high levels of vitamin B and fiber, pineapples can reduce inflammation thanks to an enzyme called bromelain.

Mushrooms

In general, mushrooms are a safe, healthy option for the renal diet, especially the shiitake variety, which are high in nutrients such as selenium, vitamin B, and manganese. They contain a moderate amount of plant-based protein, which is easier for your body to digest and use than animal proteins. Shiitake and portobello mushrooms are often used in vegan diets as a meat substitute, due to their texture and pleasant flavor.

Foods to avoid while being on the renal diet

Eating restrictions might be different depending upon your level of kidney disease. If you are in the early stages of kidney disease, you may have different restrictions as compared to those who are at the end-stage renal disease, or kidney failure. In contrast to this, people with an end-stage renal disease requiring dialysis will face different eating restrictions. Let's discuss some of the foods to avoid while being on the renal diet.

Dark-Colored Colas contain calories, sugar, phosphorus, etc. They contain phosphorus to enhance flavor, increase its life and avoid discoloration. Which can be found in a product's ingredient list. This addition of phosphorus varies depending on the type of cola. Mostly, the dark-coloured colas contain 50–100 mg in a 200-ml serving. Therefore, dark colas should be avoided on a renal diet.

Avocados are a source of many nutritious characteristics including their heart-healthy fats, fiber, and antioxidants. Individuals suffering from kidney disease should avoid them because avocados are rich in potassium. 150 grams of an avocado provides a whopping 727 mg of potassium. Therefore, avocados, including guacamole, must be avoided on a renal diet, especially if you are on parole to watch your potassium intake.

Canned Foods including soups, vegetables, and beans, are low in cost but contain high amounts of sodium due to the addition of salt to increase its life. Due to this amount of sodium inclusion in canned goods, people with kidney disease should avoid consumption. Opt for lower-sodium content with the label "no salt added". One more way is to drain or rinse canned foods, such as canned beans and tuna, could decrease the sodium content by 33–80%, depending on the product.

Brown Rice is a whole grain containing a higher concentration of potassium and phosphorus than its white rice counterpart. One cup already cooked brown rice possess about 150 mg of phosphorus and 154 mg of potassium, whereas, one cup of already cooked white rice has an amount of about 69 mg of phosphorus and 54 mg of potassium. Bulgur, buckwheat, pearled barley and couscous are equally beneficial, low-phosphorus options and might be a good alternative instead of brown rice.

Bananas are high potassium content, low in sodium, and provides 422 mg of potassium per banana. It might disturb your daily balanced potassium intake to 2,000 mg if a banana is a daily staple. Some more tropical fruits have high potassium contents as well. The only thing, pineapples, contain less potassium than other tropical fruits and can be a more suitable alternative.

Whole-Wheat Bread may harm individuals with kidney disease. But for healthy individuals, it is recommended over refined, white flour bread. White bread is recommended instead of whole-wheat varieties for individuals with kidney disease just because it has phosphorus and potassium. If you add more bran and whole grains in the bread, then the amount of phosphorus and potassium contents goes higher. For example, a 30-gram serving of whole-wheat bread contains about 57 mg of phosphorus and 69 mg of potassium, whereas, white bread contains only 28 mg of both phosphorus and potassium. Most bread and bread products contain high amounts of sodium.

Dairy products being rich in vitamins and nutrients, and a source of phosphorus and potassium. For example, 1 cup of whole milk provides 222 mg of phosphorus and 349 mg of potassium. So, consuming too many dairy products can be detrimental to bone health in those with kidney disease. If the kidneys are damaged, more phosphorus consumption can cause an accumulation of phosphorus in the blood. This will, in turn, make your bones thin and weak over time and increase the risk of bone breakage or fracture. It is significant to limit dairy intake to avoid the buildup of protein waste in the blood. Dairy alternatives like rice milk and almond milk are much lower in potassium, phosphorus, and protein than milk, making them a good substitute for milk while on a renal diet.

Oranges and Orange Juice are enriched with vitamin C content and potassium. 184 grams provides 333 mg of potassium and 473 mg of potassium in one cup of orange juice. With these calculations, oranges and orange juice must be avoided or used in a limited amount while being on a renal diet. Grapes, apples and cranberries, and their ciders or juices, are all alternatives for oranges and orange juice, as they possess low potassium contents.

Potatoes and sweet potatoes, being, the potassium-rich vegetables with 156 g contains 610 mg of potassium, whereas 114 g contains 541 mg of potassium which is relatively high. Some of the high-potassium foods, likewise potatoes and sweet potatoes, could also be soaked or leached to lessen the concentration of potassium contents. Cut them into small and thin pieces and boil those for at least 10 minutes can reduce the potassium content by about 50%. Potatoes which are soaked in a wide pot of water for as low as four hours before cooking could possess even less potassium content than those not soaked before cooking. This is known as "potassium leaching," or the "double cook Direction." A little amount of potassium could be present still in double-cooked potatoes, so it is best to look for portion control to keep potassium levels in check.

Packaged, Instant and Processed foods are a drastic provider of sodium in the diet. Among these foods, packaged, instant and pre-made meals are the most heavily processed and thus contain the higher concentration of sodium. Some of the names include frozen pizza, microwaveable foods, and instant noodles. To keep sodium intake to 2,000 mg per day is difficult if you consume highly processed foods daily. Heavily processed foods contain a large chunk of sodium, but also they are commonly lacking in nutrients as well.

Tomatoes are also high-potassium fruit that is not fit with the guidelines of a renal diet. They are served raw or stewed and are often used to make sauces. AS only one cup of tomato sauce can contain more than 900 mg of potassium. But, for those who are on a renal diet, tomatoes are a significant part of most of the dishes. Choosing an alternative to this with lower potassium concentration depends on taste choices. However, interchanging tomato sauce for a roasted red pepper sauce can be equally delicious, with the positive fact of providing less potassium per serving.

Dates, Raisins, and Prunes are common dried fruits. The phenomenon is, when fruits are dried, all of the nutrients are concentrated, including potassium. Let's understand this with an example: one cup of prunes is the alternative of 1,274 mg of potassium, which is about five times the amount of potassium found in one cup of its raw plums. Moreover, only four dates are the other name of 668 mg of potassium. With this exceptional amount of potassium found in these dried fruits, it's best to avoid while on a renal diet to ensure potassium levels remain favorable.

Snack foods like pretzels, chips, and crackers are the foods that lack nutrients and are much higher in salt. It is easy to eat more than the recommended portion size of these foods, often leading to even greater salt intake than intended. If chips, being made from potatoes, they will contain a significant amount of potassium as well.

If you are suffering from or living with kidney disease, reducing your potassium, phosphorus and sodium intake is an essential aspect of managing and tackling the disease. The foods with high-potassium, high-sodium, and high-phosphorus content listed above should always be limited or avoided. These restrictions and nutrients intakes may differ depending on the level of damage to your kidneys. Following a renal diet might be a daunting procedure and a restrictive one most of the times. But, working with your physician and nutrition specialist and a renal dietitian can assist you to formulate a renal diet specific to your individual needs.

How Eating Well Can Make a Difference

The renal diet focuses primarily on supporting kidney health because in doing so, you'll improve many other aspects of your health, as well. It can also be customized to fit all levels of kidney disease, from early stages and minor infections to more significant renal impairment and dialysis. Preventing the later stages is the main goal, though reaching this stage can still be treated with careful consideration of your dietary choices. In addition to medical treatment, the diet provides a way for you to gain control over your health and progression. It can mean the difference between a complete renal failure or a manageable chronic condition, where you can lead a regular, enjoyable life despite having kidney issues.

Eating Well is a Natural and Medicine-Free Way to Help Your Kidneys

Whether or not the medication is a part of your treatment plan, your diet takes on a significant role in the health of your kidneys. Some herbs and vitamins can boost the medicinal properties found in foods and give your kidneys additional support, while limiting other ingredients which, in excess, can lead to complete renal failure if there are already signs of kidney impairment. Your kidneys thrive on fresh, unprocessed foods that make it easier for your body to break down, digest, and process nutrients. Choosing natural options also eliminates or reduces the amount of sodium and refined sugars you consume, so you don't have to continuously monitor how many grams of salt or sugar are in your foods.

If you have limited access to fresh fruits or vegetables, choose frozen as the next best option, as they will have retained all or most of the nutrients in their original state. Canned vegetables and fruits are often processed, though these can be added when no other options are available. To reduce the amount of sodium they contain, rinse canned vegetables in the water at least twice before adding them to your meal or dish. Canned fruit is often preserved in a thick or sugary syrup, which should be drained and rinsed before serving, to reduce the sugar content. Always read the ingredients of the package or can before you consider adding it to your grocery cart, and only choose these options where fresh or frozen selections are unavailable.

Unless directed by a physician or medical specialist, don't reduce or stop taking medication for your kidneys, even if there are significant improvements to your health as a result of dietary changes and/or medical improvements, and there is an increase in kidney function noted. While diet should be a central part of your lifestyle, keep the medication as part of this treatment goal just the same. Any sudden or significant changes in your treatment plan can thwart any progress made and may cause further damage in the long term. Consider your food and meal choices in the renal diet as part of a whole, which also includes exercise, medical treatment(s), and living well.

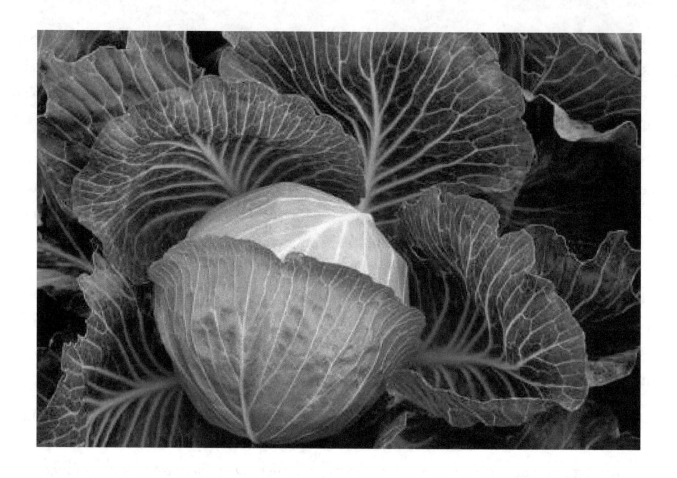

Chapter 8: Renal Diet Meal Plan

Nobody likes restrictions. And if you're used to cooking a certain way, suddenly being faced with a new list of restrictions can intimidate even the most experienced chef. You'll quickly realize that it is possible to enjoy meals—perhaps more than ever before—regardless of the recommended limitations imposed by renal complications. A basic strategy for sticking with a kidney-healthy diet is to be aware of the nutrient content in your meals and the types of nutrients you may need to limit. For example, you'll be looking to choose foods with less sodium and the right kinds of protein.

You'll see that while these rules are beneficial for slowing the progression of kidney damage, they are healthy for the general population, as well. So by all means, include your family in your health-supportive menu planning. Lowering sodium intake, for example, will decrease anyone's risk for high blood pressure, while choosing better protein options will decrease saturated fat intake for all diners and, in turn, limit the chances of developing atherosclerosis and heart disease.

To keep the body functioning properly, we all require essential macronutrients such as fat, carbohydrates, and protein, and micronutrients such as sodium and potassium. Being on the renal diet does not change this fundamental fact. However, it does alter the amounts of certain nutrients that the body can tolerate and process. For example, did you know that 1 teaspoon of table salt equals 2,300 milligrams of sodium? This is already the maximum amount a person should consume in one day!

THE LOW-SODIUM RENAL DIET MEAL PLAN

Many of the basic dietary principles on the renal diet are related to the fluid. The inability of the kidneys to excrete fluid also means that water-soluble nutrients can build up in the body and cause harmful effects. Certain nutrients, such as sodium, can cause the body to retain fluid, which can increase blood pressure and place added stress on the heart.

There are several ways to limit sodium intake while maintaining a flavorful diet. To control blood pressure, less than 2,300 milligrams of sodium (1 teaspoon) should be consumed per day. This may sound difficult if you're accustomed to keeping a saltshaker on your table, but there are plenty of substitutions that can be made for old-fashioned table salt. For example, substituting dried herbs and seasoning, such as basil and oregano, can maximize flavor without sodium (see Dump the Salt: Explore Your Options, here). Keep in mind that there may be sodium hiding in certain store-bought products, so make sure to check the nutrition labels. Also, watch out for unwanted sodium in canned or frozen foods. A simple trick is to rinse your canned vegetables or beans before eating them, which will eliminate a significant amount of the sodium from the food item. If you buy frozen dinners, look for the low-sodium varieties. But without a doubt, buying fresh, whole foods as often as possible is the best way to control what you are putting in your body.

DUMP THE SALT: EXPLORE YOUR OPTIONS

The science is clear: sodium is of no help to kidneys that are working hard already. But a little experimenting will have you kicking the salt habit as you discover flavorful alternatives that can become your new go-to seasonings. Try some of these tasty, healthier flavor boosters on your meats, grains, and veggies:

- Beer or wine (use sparingly)
- Cardamom
- Cayenne pepper
- Cilantro
- Cinnamon
- Dill
- Garlic and olive oil (just a small bit of oil will fill your dish with flavor!)
- Lemon
- Rosemary
- Scallions, leeks, onions
- Vinegar (there are countless varieties available)

Don't let the list stop here! The supermarket is packed with great fresh and dried herbs and spices. One caution: Beware of packaged salt substitutes and spice blends that may contain added salt. The best route is always to create your blend from ingredients you've chosen.

Week 1 Meal Plan

Monday

Breakfast: Blueberry Bread Pudding

Lunch: Simple Cabbage Soup

Dinner: Marinated Chicken, Grilled Zucchini and Red Onion Salad

Tuesday

Breakfast: Baked Egg Casserole

Lunch: Simple Cabbage Soup

Dinner: Stuffed Bell Peppers

Wednesday

Breakfast: Blackberry Kale Smoothie

Lunch: Cobb Salad

Dinner: Pork with Brown Sugar Rub, Peach Cucumber Salad

Thursday

Breakfast: Blueberry Citrus Muffins

Lunch: Fish Tacos with Vegetable Slaw

Dinner: Vegetable Stew

Friday

Breakfast: Pretty Pink Smoothie

Lunch: Vegetable Stew

Dinner: Homestyle Hamburgers

Saturday

Breakfast: Baked Egg Casserole

Lunch: Crunchy Chicken Salad Wraps

Dinner: Lime Baked Haddock (here), Bulgur Vegetable Salad

Sunday

Breakfast: Spiced French Toast

Lunch: Chicken Alphabet Soup

Dinner: Ginger Spiced Lamb Chops, German Braised Cabbage

Suggested Snacks

Blueberry Citrus Muffins

Citrus Sesame Cookies

Hardboiled eggs

Grapes

Unsalted popcorn

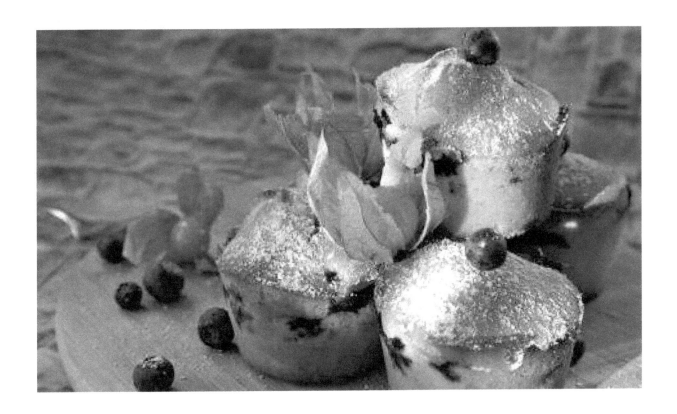

Chapter 9: How to Slow Kidney Disease

A kidney disease diagnosis can seem devastating at first. The news may come as a shock for some people, who may not have experienced any symptoms. It's important to remember that you can control your progress and improvement through diet and lifestyle changes, even when a prognosis is serious. Taking steps to improve your health can make a significant effort to slow the progression of kidney disease and improve your quality of life.

Focus on Weight Loss

Losing weight is one of the most common reasons for going on a diet. It's also one of the best ways to treat kidney disease and prevent further damage. Carrying excess weight contributes to high toxicity levels in the body, by storing toxins instead of releasing them through the kidneys. Eating foods high in trans fats, sugar, and excess sodium contribute to obesity, which affects close to one third of North Americans and continues to rise in many other countries, where fast foods are becoming easier to access and less expensive. Losing weight is a difficult cycle for many, who often diet temporarily only to return to unhealthy habits after reaching a milestone, which results in gaining the weight back, thus causing an unhealthy "yo-yo" diet effect.

There are some basic and easy changes you can make to shed those first pounds, which will begin to take the pressure off the kidneys and help you onto the path of regular weight loss:

• Drink plenty of water. If you can't drink eight glasses a day, try adding unsweetened natural sparkling water or herbal teas to increase your water intake.

• Reduce the amount of sugar and carbohydrates you consume. This doesn't require adapting to a ketogenic or low-carb diet – you'll notice a major change after ditching soda and reducing the bread and pasta by half.

• Take your time to eat and avoid rushing. If you need to eat in a hurry, grab a piece of fruit or a small portion of macadamia nuts. Avoid sugary and salty foods as much as possible. Choose fresh fruits over potato chips and chocolate bars.

• Create a short list of kidney-friendly foods that you enjoy and use this as your reference or guide when grocery shopping. This will help you stock up on snacks, ingredients, and foods for your kitchen that work well within your renal diet plan, at the same time reducing your chances of succumbing to the temptation of eating a bag of salted pretzels or chocolate.

Once you make take a few steps towards changing the way you eat, it will get easier. Making small changes at first is the key to success and to progressing with a new way of eating and living. If you are already in the habit of consuming packaged foods – such as crackers, chips, processed dips, sauces and sodas, for example – try cutting down on one or two items at a time, and over a while, gradually eliminate and cut down other items. Slowly replace these with fresh foods and healthier choices, so that your body has a chance to adapt without extreme cravings that often occur during sudden changes.

Quit Smoking and Reduce Alcohol

It's not easy to quit smoking or using recreational drugs, especially where there has been long-term use and the effects have already made an impact on your health. At some point, you'll begin to notice a difference in the way you feel and how your body changes over time. This includes chronic coughing related to respiratory conditions, shortness of breath, and a lack of energy. These changes may be subtle at first, and it may appear as though there is minimal damage or none at all, though smoking inevitably catches up with age and contributes to the development of cancer, premature aging and kidney damage. The more toxins we consume or add to our body, the more challenging it becomes for the kidneys to work efficiently, which eventually slows their ability to function.

For most people, quitting "cold turkey" or all at once is not an option, because of the withdrawal symptoms and increased chances of starting again. This method, however, can work if applied with a strong support system and a lot of determination, though it's not the best option for everyone. Reducing smoking on your own, or switching to e-cigarettes or a patch or medication, can help significantly over time. Setting goals of reduction until the point of quitting can be a beneficial way to visualize success and provide a sense of motivation. The following tips may also be useful for quitting smoking and other habit-forming substances:

• Join a support group and talk to other people who relate to you. Share your struggles, ideas, and thoughts, which will help others as well as yourself during this process.

• Track your progress on a calendar or in a notebook, either by pen and paper or on an application. This can serve as a motivator, as well as a means to display how you've done so far and where you can improve. For example, you may have reduced your smoking from ten to seven cigarettes per day, then increased to nine. This may indicate a slight change that can keep in mind to focus on reducing your intake further, from nine cigarettes to seven or six per day, and so on.

• Be aware of stressors in your life that cause you to smoke or use substances. If these factors are avoidable, make every effort to minimize or stop them from impacting your life. This may include specific people, places, or situations that can "trigger" a craving or make you feel more likely to use than usual. If there are situations that you cannot avoid, such as family, work, or school-related situations, consult with a trusted friend or someone you can confide in who can be present with you during these instances.

• Don't be afraid to ask for help. Many people cannot quit on their own without at least some assistance from others. Seeking the guidance and expertise of a counselor or medical professional to better yourself can be one of the most important decisions you make to improve the quality of your life.

Getting Active

One of the most important ways to keep fit and healthy is by staying active and engaging in regular exercise. Regular movement is key, and exercise is different for everyone, depending on their abilities and options available. Fortunately, there are unlimited ways to customize an exercise routine or plan that can suit any lifestyle, perhaps low impact to start, or if you're ready, engage in a more vigorous workout. For many people experiencing kidney disease, one of the major struggles is losing weight and living a sedentary life, where movement is generally minimal and exercise is generally not practiced. Smoking, eating processed foods, and not getting the required nutrition can further impair the body in such a way that exercise is seen as a hurdle and a challenge that is best avoided. Making lifestyle changes is not something that should be done all at once, but over a while – especially during the early stages of renal disease – so that the impact of the condition is minimized over time and becomes more manageable.

Where can you begin, if you haven't exercised at all or for a long period? For starters, don't sign up for a marathon or engage in any strenuous activities unless it is safe to do so. Start slow and take your time. Before taking on any new movements – whether it is minimal, low-impact walking or stretching, or a more moderate to the high-impact regimen – always talk to your doctor to rule out any impact this may have on other existing conditions, such as blood pressure and respiratory conditions, as well as your kidneys. Most, if not all, physicians will likely recommend exercise as part of the treatment plan but may advise beginning slowly if your body isn't used to exercise.

Simple techniques to introduce exercise into your life require a commitment. This can begin with a quick 15-minute walk or jog and a 10-or 15-minute stretch in the morning before starting your day. There are several easy, introductory techniques to consider, including the following:

• Take a walk for 10 to 15 minutes each day, at least three or four days each week. If you find it difficult at first, due to cramping, respiratory issues, or other conditions, walk slowly and breathe deeply. Make sure you feel relaxed during your walks. Find a scenic path or area in your neighborhood that is pleasant and gives you something to enjoy, such as a beautiful sunset or forested park. Bring a bottle of water to keep yourself hydrated.

• Stretch for five minutes once a day. This doesn't mean you need to do any intricate yoga poses or specific techniques. Moving your ankles, wrists, and arms in circles and standing every so often (if you sit often) and twisting your torso can help release stress and improve your blood flow, which lowers blood pressure and helps your body transport nutrients to areas in need of repair.

• Practice breathing long, measured breaths. This will help prepare you for more endurance-based exercise, such as jogging, long walks, cycling, and swimming. Count to five on each inhale and exhale, and practice moving slowly as you breathe, to "sync" or coordinate your body's movements with your breathing. If you have difficulty with the respiratory system, take it slow and don't push yourself. If you feel weak or out of breath, stop immediately and try again later or the next day at a slower pace.

• Start a beginner's yoga class and learn the fundamentals of various poses and stretches. It is helpful to arrive early and speak with the instructor, who can provide guidance on which modifications work best if needed. They may also be able to provide tips on how to approach certain poses or movements that can be challenging for beginners so that you feel more comfortable and knowledgeable before you start.

• If you smoke, exercise will present more of a challenge on your lungs and respiratory function. Once you become accustomed to a beginner's level and become moderately active, you may notice it takes more effort, which requires an increase in lung capacity and oxygen. Smoking will eventually present a challenge, and where quitting can be a long-term and difficult goal in itself, make an effort to cut back as much as it takes to allow your body's movements and exercise continue. In time, you may find quitting becomes easier and more achievable than expected!

Once you get into a basic routine, there is a wide variety of individual and team activities to consider for your life. If you are a social person, joining a baseball team or badminton club may be ideal. For more solitary options, consider swimming, cycling, or jogging. Many gyms and community centers provide monthly plans and may offer a free trial period to see if their facilities work for you. This is a great opportunity to try new classes and equipment to gauge how much you can achieve, even if in the early stages of exercise so that you can decide whether to pursue dance aerobics, spin classes and/or weight training. Some gyms will provide a free consultation with a personal trainer to set a simple plan towards weight loss and strength training goals.

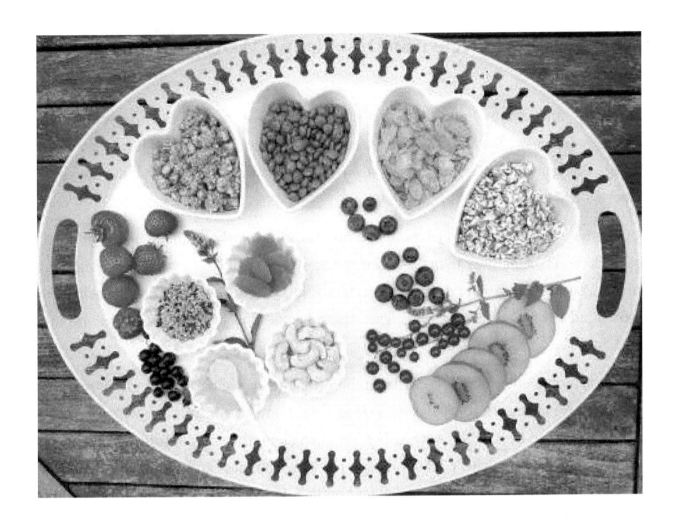

Chapter 10: The Reasons Diets Don't Work

The energy and money that Americans spend each year wanting to lose weight could practically run a small country! The cost of overweight human discontent is incalculable. There is a reason why Americans are still overweight although they spend all this weight loss money... diets don't work!

However, it is important to understand first how the mind works to understand why diets do not work. You'll be halfway to make major changes in your life until you understand how it works... You will change your destiny if you change your mind! There are three principal areas of the mind I will discuss... the conscious, the subconscious, and the critical sphere of the mind.

Our short-term memory is the conscious mind. It is the logical part of the mind, reasoning, and decision-making. Here we decide to lose weight, and it controls our willpower in our brain. We need to be conscious of the need to change, motivated to improve and to believe that we can achieve our goal to make positive changes and become mentally fit. Consciousness is the responsible component of the mind. It accounts for around 12% of our brain capacity.

Our long-term memory is the unconscious mind. It represents the remaining 88 percent and always hears, always watches, and is eagerly awaiting instructions on how to help. It is the most powerful computer that has ever been created, able to run several tasks at the same time. We don't evaluate, condemn, examine, or deny... we just record and respond. He doesn't understand; he doesn't have a sense of humor and takes it all.

But there is hope.... if we want to change a behavior, we have to "hack in" the unconscious and change the existing system of belief (reprogramming the operating system). We do this by Hypnosis.

How many times have you tried to do something that needed the power of will, only to fail? This doesn't mean you're weak. You see, the conscious mind, from which willpower and reason come, uses only about 12% of our brain-power. The remaining 88% comes from the subconscious.

For example, because diets do not work, they rely on the conscious mind. Remember, only about 12 percent of your mind makes up the conscious mind, where we get our willpower. The subconscious, the part that constitutes the other 88%, fights against it! It's so hard to lose weight, no wonder! When 88% of your mind says yes to chocolate cake, it will make it difficult for poor little 12% of your mind to combat it.

Let me give you another example. Perhaps for many years, you have been overweight, and you decide that it's a new year. It's time you finally started your diet and made it stick. However, if you consciously decide to lose weight, you only use the conscious area of your mind (12%). Your subconscious (88 percent) believes that you have always been overweight, tried, and failed many times with a wide variety of different diets, and you will never be thin. For the unconscious, you were always overweight, you were always overweight, and you could not do or do anything to change it!

Hypnosis can be very helpful here. While the critical mind is hypnotized, it allows the subconscious mind to open up and accept positive suggestions (such as turning off the spam filter to allow a specific program to download to your hard drive). This allows us to "download" new suggestions into your subconscious to change your thinking and to create an image that is always thin at a healthier weight so that you can achieve your goals!

So what does all this mean in terms of diet and weight loss? It's really, very simple. When a suggestion is "downloaded" in the subconscious mind, it is a "known fact." We often use self-suggestion in our daily lives, often without even realizing it. You see, everything has to do with the way we see ourselves. Statements or thoughts like "I can't lose weight, no matter how hard I try" or "I'm never going to be able to do that" are very powerful but very negative. (Remember that the subconscious takes all literally, and whether or not it is true, considers it to be a' fact') Our subconscious mind is innocent and naive. It tries to protect and help us and tries to the best of its ability. But the intelligence level of about a four-year-old child often doesn't serve us the right way and needs to be diverted.

Hypnosis comes in here. Hypnotherapy is a highly effective way to manage problems such as being overweight. Hypnotherapy In Hypnosis, we suggest "you can lose weight" and "you will be able to do so." Statistics show that Hypnosis can significantly increase not only the chances of losing excess weight, but also keeps it healthy.

Naturally, Hypnosis works only if you do your part. Like any training program, you actually have to be the one to do the job. As the saying goes, you can't pay anyone to push you! The hypnotherapist does not do hypnosis "to you." Your mind is like a muscle. Your mind. You must practice it. The job of the hypnotist is like a personal trainer, guiding you, and helping you to achieve your objective. You can go to the fitness room seven days a week, but if your personal trainer lifts all your weights, your muscles don't grow taller. Your hypnotherapist can help and motivate you with guided imagery and other techniques, but you still have to make an effort to succeed.

Certain procedures appear to produce very reliable positive results. In Hypnosis, we suggest that you can still eat what you like, but that you reduce the amount of food you eat. By taking good care of yourself, your mind and body start working together more and more. Using Hypnosis and following these simple instructions, you will lose excess weight and stay away from it for the rest of your life.

Below is a list of things you can do to guarantee your success: 1. If you have to lose more than 20-30 pounds, a physical exam is always a good idea before you begin a weight loss program.

2. Request a sensible, balanced diet plan from your doctor. Hypnotherapy aims to restructure your diet so that you not only lose weight but also retain it by maintaining a sensible eating pattern for the rest of your life. Avoid crash and faded diets! You may lose weight, but you will not establish a permanent eating pattern to keep it away.

3. Planning to lose up to 2 pounds a week. This reduces the physical strain to a minimum, reduces your feelings of urgency and anxiety, and allows you to adapt to your new self. Two pounds a week may not seem like a lot now, but you could have been 100 pounds lighter one year from now if you follow that plan! (And how much in a year will you weigh if you decide to do what you did?) 4. Do not worry if you can achieve deep hypnosis or not. Sometimes

lighter-state subjects appear to have better effects than deeper-state subjects on weight therapy.

5. Consider the times of day when you have the most difficulty resisting food problems and attempt to replace some other activity or think of unwanted food patterns. You could go for a walk, for example. It would drive you away from the source of the food you crave and potentially provide you with a good workout.

6. Don't be a disincentive. Some people can eat up for seven days and only lose a pound. However, they may lose 3 inches simultaneously since their fatty deposits can become liquid, and liquid weighs 12% more than fat. Weigh yourself only once a week to minimize depression.

In weight therapy, your motivation must be constantly stimulated because lasting results are achieved gradually. Therefore, in our weight management program, we use reinforcement CDs, which should be heard every night about 30 minutes before bedtime. Hearing them every night will help keep you on track for the duration of the program. It is also crucial to continue learning about your new eating patterns, physicality, and self-esteem. Ultimately, the things you learned will motivate and strengthen new eating patterns.

Renal Failure and Proper Nutrition

The kidneys are twin organs that filter the blood to remove all waste products. The kidneys often start releasing blood pressure hormones and red blood cell count. The blood enters the kidneys, and the waste is diverted and sent via the ureter into the bladder so that in the act of urination, it is removed from the body. The filtered blood goes back to the body. In total, over eighteen blood of gallons are filtered every hour for the kidney for a total of 432 gallons of blood. The kidneys also filter more than half of the body's fluids and release at least two-quarters of urine every day.

The kidneys may be subjected to a range of different disorders, including kidney infections, kidney stones, and a severe condition called chronic renal disease (CKD).

Renal failure can be acute or chronic, usually detected by increased serum creatinine and decreased glomerular filtration. Renal failure may have several symptoms including: — increased blood urea levels— Dehydration— Missile — Weight loss— Night urination— Foamy or urine bubbly — Increased frequency or increases in the amounts of pale urine— urine blood — pressure or urine difficulty Renal failure may also lead to phosphates. Hypertension, particularly when not treated, gout, diabetes, prolonged impacts, and the use of certain drugs, are some of the risk factors for kidney disease.

The chronic renal disease affects 26 million Americans, and millions more are at high risk for the disease. Early detection is essential to ensure that CKD does not lead to renal failure. Heart disease is the leading cause of death for CKD patients. Hypertension is an important risk factor for CKD, but CKD is also an important risk factor for hypertension development. Both can be called interchangeable because they are so connected. Virtually everyone with CKD will have high blood pressure, and most people with hypertension are more likely to develop CKD.

Other risk factors include higher blood pressure: diabetes, a family history of kidney disease, and certain ethnic groups. African, Hispanic, Pacific Islander, or Native American people are at increased risk of these and other kidney diseases.

Causes of Kidney Disease: -Hypovolemia (low blood volume) can be the result of extreme blood loss-dehydration — diuretic use— Renal artery or vein obstruction.

Sepsis-Trauma or crushing accidents - Rhabdomyolyses (important muscle breakdown in the body) - diseases that affect the kidney may be temporary or potentially fatal. Therapy can be as simple as medicines or as complex as the need for a new kidney. If one of them happens, it's never a good idea to do so when you can survive with only one kidney, because it puts so much pressure on the remaining organ. Three common tests are conducted to check for kidney failure, including blood pressure, urine albumin, and serum creatinine. High blood pressure may be a symptom of kidney disease because the kidneys secrete blood pressure hormones.

Everyone with a chronic condition of any kind should seek advice on nutrition and the need for vitamins and minerals from his / her doctor. Many micronutrients may be detrimental to the already overtaxed body. Certain macronutrients may be harmful to people with CKD or other kidney problems.

People with CKD should restrict their intake of protein within a reasonable period only under the guidance and direction of a nutritionist (Source: National Clearing House for Urological and Kidney Disease). Protein is an important part of a healthy diet, but for those with kidney disease, certain restrictions exist. The amount of protein may be important to limit so that the protein you receive should be of high quality and low fat.

Too much protein in the diet changes the metabolism process into a ketosis state. Ketosis happens when the body stops burning energy with carbohydrates and instead returns to fat. The fat is divided into carbon molecules called ketones. These ketones are released into the flow of blood.

Ketosis can be problematic as appetite is suppressed while urinary efficiency is increased. The American Heart Association suggests that the amount of protein in the diet is no greater than 35 percent of daily calories, but that this can be much too much for those suffering from early or deteriorating kidney disease. The combination can lead to dehydration, electron imbalance, and osteoporosis (source: Osterweil). It is important to ensure that physicians and nutritionists work to find the correct number of macronutrients, protein, fat, and carbohydrates that work with kidney disease. The proteins eaten should be healthy, low-fat, including plant proteins.

In addition to the above-mentioned severe kidney conditions, kidney stones also exist. One of the most painful urological conditions is kidney stones. It is also one of the most frequent. Although most of the kidney stones a person develops pass without medical intervention, some people may need to be treated.

Calcium oxalate or the phosphate oxalate stone with a few other, less common types of stones are the most common type. Kidney stones in Caucasian men between 40 and 70 years of age are the most common. The threat of kidney stones in women reaches the age of 50 years.

Your chances of kidney stones rise family history, frequent UTIs, cystic kidney disease, and some metabolic disorders. Cystinuria and hyperoxaluria are both rare metabolism disorders that are inherited and can cause renal stones in many cases. Also inherited is hypercalciuria (high calcium in the blood), which can cause half of the kidney stones. Other causes: gout, vitamin D surplus, urinary tract blockage, and diuretic use.

Kidney Stone symptoms— There are several symptoms: extreme pain, sharp back pain, nausea and vomiting, pink urine, frequent urination, urination burns, chills, fever. In the course of excluding additional conditions, most kidney stones are found by an X-ray, CT scan, or intravenous pyelogram.

The Rest of the Diet Equation

The fact that the abdominal definition of the abdominal system is as straightforward as following a healthy diet can disappoint anyone who wants to follow the latest buzz routine, but the truth is that there are no miracle exercises, machines or tablets that give you the abs you want unless your diet is proper. As the saying goes, "healthy abs are done not in the gym in the kitchen."

Furthermore, the good news here is that if you know that a healthy food plan is key to your success, it is very easy for you to use this knowledge. Why? Why? Because unlike the enormous muscles of someone such as Arnold Schwarzenegger or the strength of the world's strongest men, everyone can achieve a great abdominal definition regardless of their genetic characteristics, age, or current weight. The reality is that if you follow the correct healthy eatery and education program for long enough, you'll get a perfect six-pack, and that's a scientific fact. So what is a healthy eating plan? The solution is always right for you, and by that, I don't mean the break-out of the hobnobs (sorry) I mean that you have fewer calories to consume than your body needs.

How many calories do you know you need?

A variety of rough guides are available to measure the rate of calorie maintenance. One way is to add a weight of 15 (for men) or 12 (for women) to your body (in pounds). For example, a man of 140 pounds (15x140) = 2100 calories a day would be needed to keep his weight. However, it is important to remember that many other factors, such as your metabolic rate, muscle mass level, age, and also your overall level of activity, must be considered. It is, therefore, unlikely for such a guide to be 100% accurate, but it will give you an idea.

The next step is to figure out exactly how many calories you eat from the food you eat. This can be done by simply taking notice for several days of the weight and nutritional data on food labels. Once you have done this, you should know how many calories you eat. Now that you know how many calories you eat to maintain the same weight, your intake should be reduced by 500 days and how your body reacts. You will lose about 1 pound of fat a week if you have correctly estimated your calorie maintenance and then lower your daily intake to 500 calories a day, as there are 4000 calories in one pound of fat.

The goal of 1-pound weekly weight loss is most likely, and although you can increase it to 2 pounds per week if you are impatient, do not exceed that level as if you are losing almost as much muscle mass as you do fat, which is never a good idea. Therefore, once you begin your healthy diet, take all your measures, weigh yourself once a week, and look at your body in the mirror to see if you progress steadily.

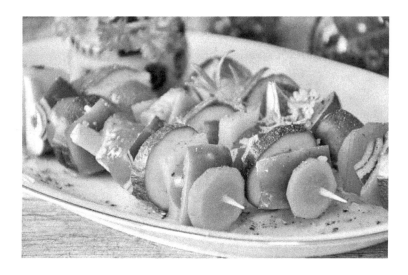

Chapter 11: The Basics of Renal Diet

1.   Eat good quality and the right amounts of protein

Limited portions

You need to limit the amount of protein you consume. Why? This is because you need to help protect the kidneys by reducing their workload. The thing is; when the body uses protein to produce energy, it produces a lot of waste. More protein means more waste and thus more work.

Why does it need to be from high-quality sources?

Forget protein shakes and other processed forms of protein. Eat quality proteins from plants and animals to meet your dietary needs. Low-quality protein will not give you the sufficient nutrients you need and it will increase the amount of toxic waste in the body.

Quality protein sources

- Quality animal protein foods include; lamb, poultry, beef and fish. You can also have eggs and milk products and low phosphorous cheese such as cottage, goat or brie cheese.
- Plant sources of protein; legumes, soya, nuts and grains.

2.   Choose and prepare foods with less sodium

Sodium is widely used in food preparation. It is important to note that salt and sodium are not interchangeable; salt is made of sodium but sodium is not salt.

Let me explain.

Salt is a compound of sodium and chloride. Some use table salt while others will contain other forms of sodium, especially those used in seasoning and preserving most canned and processed foods.

It is important to reduce the amount of sodium consumed for the sake of your blood pressure. According to experts, too much sodium in the blood will increase it to a point where it becomes unhealthy.

Purposes of sodium in the body

This compound is one of the body's major electrolytes. The function of sodium in the body is to control the fluids going in and out of the body. Other than fluid control, sodium helps with the following functions:

- Regulating the acid-base balance in the blood
- Regulating blood pressure and blood volume
- Regulation of nerve functions and muscle contraction

We need sodium but at low levels. Too much of it will wreak havoc in the body.

Why should kidney patients keep track of their sodium intake?

When you have kidney disease, these bean-shaped organs will not be able to adequately remove sodium and fluid from the body. When sodium and fluid build up in the body, it can result in:

- High blood pressure (as mentioned earlier)
- Shortness of breath as fluid can build up in the lungs, making it hard to breathe.
- Increased thirst
- Edema; swelling in the legs, face and hands
- Heart failure as excess fluid in your bloodstream could end up overworking your heart, enlarging it and making it weak.

How to ensure that you are ingesting less sodium

- Carefully read food labels. Some foods are not necessarily salty but they contain lots of sodium. Look for labels such as salt-free or sodium-free, unsalted or slightly salted.

- Buy fresh foods to eat and prepare in the kitchen. You want to avoid canned and ready to eat foods which are often high in sodium.
- In place of salt, use herbs and sodium-free spices and seasonings to make your food tasty.
- If you have to use canned foods such as vegetables, beans, fish or meat, rinse them with water before cooking to get rid of the excess traces of sodium.
- Cook your meals from scratch. This way, you can control how much salt goes into it compared to if you are having to take away and pre-prepared frozen food.
- Limit sodium to 400mg per meal and at most 150mg per snack

3.   Maintain the right potassium levels in the body

Potassium is greatly involved in the functioning of body muscles and keeping the heartbeat regular. The right amounts of this mineral will help your nerves and muscles to work properly. This is very important because there will be problems if potassium levels in the blood are either too high or too low.

The kidneys are responsible for maintaining the levels of this mineral in the blood and they will expel excess amounts in urine.

When they are not working properly, Potassium will build up in the blood and it becomes a toxic substance. This causes changes in the heartbeat and could lead to a heart attack.

How to ensure you are eating just the right amounts of potassium

It is important to note that most potassium comes from dairy products, vegetables and fruits. You may need to choose carefully and limit the consumption of such foods. However, you also need to eat some potassium rich foods to ensure that you have not completely cut it out like this, as mentioned before, could also lead to serious health problems.

Foods higher in potassium to avoid

- All kinds of dried beans
- Grapefruit juice

- Cooked leafy greens such as spinach, kales and Swiss chards
- Oranges and orange juice
- Tomatoes and tomato juice
- Bananas
- Brown rice
- Pasta and whole wheat bread
- All kinds of potatoes
- Nuts, seed and lentils

Foods low in potassium to consider (eat with moderation)

- Apples
- Grapes
- White rice and white bread
- Carrots
- Green beans
- Peaches

Note:

- You could soak and drain legumes before cooking to greatly reduce the amount of potassium they contain.
- Also, many low-sodium foods, which you may go for to keep your sodium consumption low contain added potassium chloride, which you want to avoid. Therefore, read labels carefully and watch out for this mineral.

4.   Keep phosphorus on the low

Phosphorus is important in the maintenance of healthy bones and blood vessels. The kidneys are responsible for filtering out excesses of this mineral in the blood.

Why kidney patients should monitor their intake of phosphorus

However, when the kidneys are not working properly, it will build up in the blood and become harmful.

Too much phosphorus in the blood may lead to the pulling of calcium from the bones and have it collect in the skin and blood vessels. This will result in thin, weakened and easy to break bones and also itchy skin and joint pain. Also, these dangerous calcium deposits may find their way to the lungs, eyes and heart and cause damage.

How to ensure that you are ingesting low amounts of phosphorus

- Notice the label "PHOS" on ingredient labels and avoid such products.
- When choosing protein, it is important to know that some deli meats have added phosphorus to keep it fresh. Therefore, always ask the butchers to help you choose naturally fresh pieces – they would know better.
- Avoid processed foods as they contain high amounts of inorganic phosphate.
- Limit dairy foods, which tend to be high in this mineral and replace them with un-enriched rice and soy alternatives.
- Avoid dark colored sodas and canned/bottled ice teas and instead, go for light-colored sodas and homemade iced tea.
- Eat fresh fruits and vegetables in moderation.
- Cut out beer – all kinds contain phosphorus.

5. Choose heart-healthy foods

You want to keep fat from building up in your blood vessels, the heart and kidneys. Therefore, eat foods that are not adding too much fat in the body. Also, prepare foods in such a way that there are not too much-added fats.

How to prepare heart-friendly meals

- Trim fat from meat and remove the skin from poultry before cooking
- Instead of butter, prepare your foods with small amounts of olive oil or non-stick cooking oil

- Avoid deep frying foods. Instead, cook by grilling, boiling, baking, roasting or simply stir-fry foods.

Heart-healthy food choices

- Fish
- Loa fat milk and cheese
- Vegetables
- Fruits
- Lean cuts of meat
- Legumes

6.   Limit your alcohol intake

It would be best if you avoided alcohol completely especially if you have kidney diseases – you do not want to add the extra work, do you?

However, if you have to, take it in moderation. This means no more than 1 bottle per day as a woman and not more than two for a man. These amounts are considered healthy and anything exceeding that could lead to damage of the liver, heart and brain and also increase the likelihood of having visceral fat (fat stored around the abdomen) which could lead to a myriad of health complications.

7.   Limiting of fluids

No, you cannot wake up and decide to limit your fluids because you read it here or anywhere else. For this, you are going to need expert advice from a specialist – after a series of tests.

It is important to understand that fluid restriction is a recommendation that comes only from your doctor. You do not want to restrict fluid when you should be taking it as this could lead to more problems. Therefore, take enough fluids until the doctor advises otherwise.

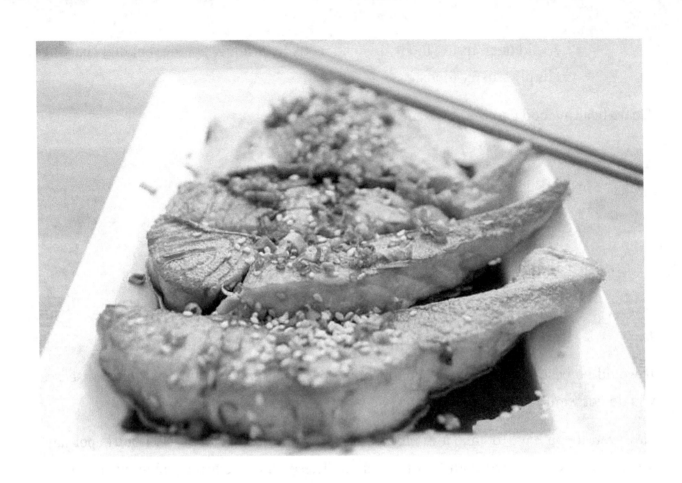

Chapter 12: Eating Well To Live Well

One of the biggest issues that they have realized that the fast foods that were once advertised as healthy are no longer healthy anymore. Most individuals had fallen for the idea that processed snacks were a convenient option for them since they were busy at work. However, with the increasing rates of obesity and weight-related health complications, people are more sensitized about their health and wellbeing. If you are not hitting the gym today, there is a good chance that you are on a diet. Are you one among those people who have tried all sorts of fad diets and nothing seems to work? Well, you are not alone. With numerous health concerns surrounding what people eat, Americans and the rest of the world have considered going for healthy food alternatives since they help in lowering killer diseases such as type 2 diabetes and heart disease.

The Centers for Disease Control and Prevention points out that obesity is not only common, but it is also serious and costly to the economy. Between 2015 and 2016, there were approximately 93.3 million U.S. adults who were obese (Adult Obesity Facts, 2019). Medical costs for those who are obese were also soaring in 2008 hitting approximately $150 billion. The numbers tell it all. They are a true depiction of how people are suffering simply because of unhealthy lifestyle choices that they make.

Looking at the bright side, if you have been diagnosed with prediabetes, then you are lucky. 90% of people who have prediabetes are not aware that they are suffering. Unfortunately, their unawareness could pose serious complications since it is likely that these folks will continue with their unhealthy habits. Therefore, it is safe to say that you have an opportunity to turn things around only if you decide to eat well to live a better life.

What does it mean to eat well and live well? Here's a closer look:

The Simple Art of Eating Well

Living a healthy life is simple. The only problem is that most people make a big deal out of it and they end up developing a negative attitude about a healthy life. Let's walk you through a typical day when you choose to live healthily.

In the morning, you find yourself waking up 20 minutes before your alarm goes off. This does not irritate you because you have recently been getting enough rest that your body requires. To start your day on a positive note, you take about 10 minutes to meditate while using positive affirmations to motivate you to live a healthy and happy life. Unsweetened coffee is your preferred breakfast beverage, so you take a few minutes to prepare it. The good news is that preparing your breakfast at home is more convenient since you end up saving yourself a couple of dollars instead of eating out. You crack two eggs as your ideal source of proteins. You top this with a few sliced tomatoes and chopped bell peppers. Without wasting time, you scramble your ingredients on a heated pan with olive oil. After having your breakfast, you grab a fresh fruit from the fridge and dash out to work.

A few hours later, in the midmorning, you notice that you are hungry. With your healthy eating mentality, you choose to snack on a handful of nuts. These are just enough to keep you satiated until your next meal.

During lunchtime, you take out your pre-packed lunch as you knew that you wanted to avoid the idea of eating out. Your second meal of the day contains lentils and brown rice that is topped with a salad with some little olive oil. You also remember to carry some berries to eat after your meal. After that, you take a glass of water before proceeding with your everyday routine at work.

Your nicely chosen meal will keep you satiated until the next meal, but you decide to snack on natural yogurt just to make sure that your sugar levels remain in check.

After work, you will be glad that you spent the rest of the day without eating junk food or drinking any sweetened juices. Your happy mood with motivates you to pass by the nearest gym to your home and workout for a few minutes before rushing home. After working out for 45 minutes, you are more than psyched up since you will be having a sweet potato with chicken, asparagus, and broccoli. This is the perfect meal to crown your healthy day with a smile.

Looking at the example provided, there is nothing complicated with living a good life. When was the last time you spent the entire day eating healthy foods and ensuring that you exercised? Maybe this is something that you haven't done for ages and that is could be one of the reasons why you have prediabetes. However, it is worth noting that with the meal plans and recipes that this guide will provide you, you can eat well and live well for as long as you want.

There are plenty of changes that the food landscape has gone through. People are no longer patient to prepare a meal for themselves. Often, they will opt to settle for convenient, processed foods. This is quite different from what our ancestors used to eat. Considering the rise in obesity and weight-related complications, food and our lifestyle choices are to be blamed for the killer diseases that are haunting our communities. People were genetically born to eat foods rich in nutrients, whole foods such as veggies, proteins, fruits, nuts, etc. Processed foods came along the way and destroyed the good health that people once enjoyed.

Moderation: Key to Success or Harm?

Today, we live in a world where you can access information at the touch of a button. The advent of the internet has transformed the way people access information. In terms of health, people are more informed now more than ever on the dangers of processed foods. Individuals have a clear understanding that the foods being marketed are not healthy. Marketing is just a way of luring people into eating more of these foods and avoiding healthier options. But, why do people still fall for these temptations despite their diverse knowledge about health?

Foods that are high in calories with high-fat content will not lead to good health. Sometimes we choose to snack on these dishes by consoling ourselves that we will avoid them next time. Usually, this is the beginning of our downfall as we find ourselves eating these foods more often than not. Today you might use your family gathering as an excuse to eat unhealthy dishes. The conscious decisions that we make during such times have its consequences. If you are on holiday making such decisions will lead to a slippery slope. Before you know it, you have thrown away all the health accomplishments that you have achieved for the past three or four months.

The reality of the matter is that the contents of the processed foods have an impact on our brain as it stimulates it to crave for them. This happens in the same way that you will be addicted to alcohol and other drugs. The pleasure gained from these foods excites our brains and that is why you can't stay away from them. Sooner or later, you will notice that you crave for more of the processed foods just to be satisfied in a special way that other healthier foods do not provide you.

Ever wondered why most folks will claim that they can't avoid unhealthy processed foods? A good number of them find it impossible to go for two days without snacking on foods that are high in sugar, salt, and fat. Let's be honest with ourselves, these foods are meant to keep us hooked. It's no wonder you will find yourself craving for them. The addictive component of fast foods has contributed a lot to an emotional attachment that people have with these foods. To steer away from these behaviors, we must identify our weaknesses and establish strategies that help us not to allow cravings to get the best of us.

All that being said, the family gatherings, date nights, and holidays often tempt us to choose unhealthy foods that we might not have ordinarily eaten when following a healthy meal plan. How do you go about this? The best way of overcoming temptations from these unhealthy food choices is by consciously realizing that you have the power to make the right choice regarding your health. Accordingly, the next time you eat unhealthy foods knowingly, know that you are not cheating anybody. Each decision you make has an impact on your overall health.

Eating well is like investing. Your savings account will look healthy if you make several deposits without withdrawals. Your savings account will grow faster if you continue making frequent deposits and ensure that you avoid withdrawals. In the same way, eating the right foods frequently and steering away from unhealthy foods, the faster you will attain your health goals.

At this point, you might be concerned about the foods that you wanted to eat in moderate amounts such as cookies, cake, and pizza, among other indulgence dishes. Dealing with moderation is not easy. This is something that we have to be honest about. Individuals should take a personal approach to address this matter. In this case, you should take time to determine the indulgence foods that trend to lure you to eat more of them. Indeed, we have our lists. It could be buggers, chocolates, French fries or the energy drinks that you love most. Also, we should take time to comprehend the circumstances that drive us to overindulge in these processed foods. Maybe you eat more of these foods when you are stressed or it's just the social settings that drive you to consume more.

The point is that we must understand that we can also get satisfied with healthy food options. Processed foods have blinded us from realizing that healthy foods can also satisfy us. The best part is that you not only enjoy a healthy meal, but you also avoid complications associated with unhealthy eating. Instead of resorting to binge eating when you are going through a rough patch, you should seek for emotional support. Talk to your friends about your situation and inform them that you are prone to overeating when you are not feeling good. They can help you keep off these foods. You don't have to be ashamed of sharing your feelings. It's a depiction that you are committed to living healthily.

That said, you should be cautious with the notion of moderation. Processed foods are addictive. There is a good chance that you might struggle to try to eat these foods in moderate amounts. An ideal way of dealing with these foods to understand your weaknesses. Which foods do you often crave for? With this understanding, you will be better placed to make smart choices about the foods you should eat and those you should avoid.

Creating a Better Nutritional Plan

Eating well to live well centers around the idea of resolving to make the right choices of the foods that you should eat. The important thing is that you choose foods that guarantee you live a happier and more fulfilling life.

You are what you eat. Food defines your life in profound ways. What you eat will influence how you feel about yourself. Food also determines how you age. Food will also determine whether you are at risk of certain diseases such as prediabetes, type 2 diabetes or heart disease. Therefore, food plays a crucial role in our lives. Food is life.

In a word, by adopting a healthy nutritional plan, we can dramatically change our lives. More specifically, we can enhance our health and wellbeing. The truth is that this is a sustainable approach to making sure that you live a happy life without having to indulge in fad diets. Providing your body with all the required nutrients from real food around you promotes your overall well-being and guarantees that you can lose weight naturally. Eating well is indeed a powerful secret to a happy life.

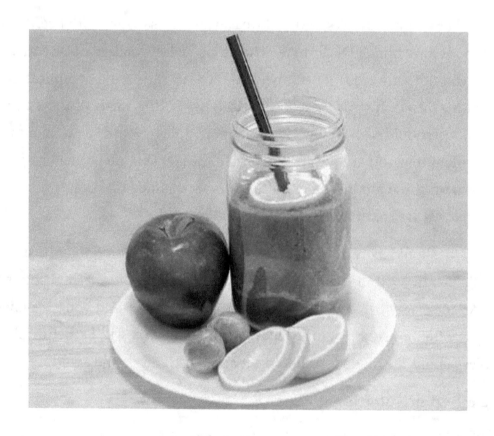

Chapter 13: Pointers to Remember When Slow Cooking

Slow cookers are safe and easy to use. It's as simple as preparing ingredients, securing the lid, turning on the machine, and setting the timer. Once you've done all those necessary steps then you're good to go, literally.

Gone are the days when you have to watch over the whole process of cooking or stir the contents of the pot often. Using a slow cooker lets you leave it overnight, so you can warm the dish the next day, or leave it while you go to work during the day, so it will be ready when you get home. You can also prepare large volumes of dishes during weekend sans slaving hours in the kitchen.

The slow cooker also uses approximately 15 to 30 watts per hour.

When using the slow cooker for the first time, it is important to take note of the following:

1. Different machines have different setting.

Models vary greatly. Some slow cooker models do not have buttons or settings. All you have to do is plug it and leave your dish to cook on its own. These machines are usually pre-set on medium heat. Therefore, if you are using this kind of model, make sure that you lessen the cooking time for dishes recommended on low heat and then extend the cooking time for recipes recommended on high heat setting.

If the "warm" function is available. Always ensure that you automatically shift to "warm mode". But regardless of your slow cooker has this function or not, your dish remains warm for up to 2 hours after cooking time.

2. All ingredients must be thawed well before cooking.

If you are using frozen veggies or meat, make sure to put them at the lower part of the fridge to drain all liquids before placing inside the slow cooker. Doing so will allow the ingredient/s to keep heat constant and prevent food to retain too much moisture.

3. Add plenty of liquids.

This is another vital rule when you are slow cooking. You would need to fill the crockpot of at least three-quarters up to prevent ingredients from sticking to the bottom of the pan. This will also prevent liquids from boiling over, which could potentially damage the machine. If the dishes have sauces, this is, of course, an exception. Make sure to adjust the volume of the liquid accordingly.

4. Take note of ingredients that are only meant to be added one hour or half an hour at the end of the cooking cycle time or oftentimes, before serving the dish.

There are also food items that only require residual heat to cook through.

Knowing about this will help prevent your food from losing texture, flavor, color, and even avoid boiling over. Also, when dealing with seafood, it is best that you only add them at the last hour or stage of cooking, or else, you'll end up serving soggy fish or dried up shellfish.

5. Some dishes would require pre-cooking.

Why is this necessary, you might ask? This is because food tastes a lot better when lightly seared or browned first. Some of them include chicken, pork, and beef.

The practice of browning meat helps enhance the depth of flavor, which means you can get more flavor out of the ingredients instead of relying on seasonings to do their job of flavoring the dish. And since this eBook is meant for people with kidney problems, this step is of greater importance especially since you will be taking out salt off the list of seasonings.

You will also notice that some recipes require the sautéing of aromatics such as onion, garlic, and ginger in a skillet before slow cooking. This is another vital step in making your dishes more flavorful. Although some slow cooker models have a "saute" function, it is still recommended that you do the sautéing in a separate skillet so you will have control over the heat.

Sautéing in a separate pan will also help you prepare for other ingredients of the recipes that would require deglazing or even those garnishes that you put on top of the dish just before serving. Some of the examples include toasted garlic, bacon bits, or even eggs, etc.

6. Let your meals cook uninterrupted.

When cooking, most people have the habit of removing the lid, stirring ingredients, and visually checking on the food from time to time. If you are going to use a slow cooker, this will not be necessary at all. Let your food be cooked undisturbed, or at least for the first 2-4 hours of cooking time before stirring.

When you make use of the slow cooker, remember to secure the lid and avoid lifting it as this may cause the temperature to drop drastically, or worse, cause injuries and accidents. If you can't stop yourself from virtually checking what you're cooking from time to time, purchase a slow cooker that has glass lids where you can easily peer into.

7. Season your meals before serving.

There are some food items such as bone-in beef, ham knuckles, potatoes, carrots, and sweet potatoes that can release or retain more flavor after cooking for a longer period.

On the other hand, you also have to be mindful of food items that tend to lose their flavor and taste after they are cooked for more than 20 minutes. Some of them include seafood, shellfish, lemon, fish, lime, and tamarinds.

Finally, seasoning before serving your cooked meals will help you gauge the taste of the food. Seasoning before cooking only gives you more reason to add more flavorings and seasonings in the process. So to ensure that you don't end up with overly salty food, season after you have turned off the slow cooker or just before serving meals.

8. A squeeze of lemon or lime will do the trick for leftover food.

Some say that slow-cooked meals are at their best taste a day or two in the freezer. To keep your dishes tastier when you reheat them, add a few drops of lime or lemon to help stimulate the taste. For sweet meals, adding a pinch of sugar will make it taste better after reheating. For spicy food, adding minced chillies will make the dish more flavorful and hot.

9. Always garnish your food. Garnish your dishes with fresh herbs, spices, fruits or vegetables.

When you use the slow cooker, there are some food items or ingredients that turn dull and become two shades darker. So to make them at least pleasing to the eyes, always remember to garnish with freshly chopped herbs and spices, fruits, vegetables, cheese, and even nuts. This will help make the dishes more enticing to eat and visually appealing. Try garnishing with vibrantly colored spices such as Spanish paprika and fresh chilies among others.

You can also try serving your dish with colorful side dishes such as carrots, corn, peas, lettuce, or lemon wedges.

10. When it comes to washing and cleaning the slow cooker, make sure to allow the machine to completely cool down at room temperature before washing.

This is particularly helpful in prolonging the life of your machine. Immediately washing it with cold water will cause the machine to crack and the metal to warp. The best time to wash the slow cooker is at least 2 hours. Should some food items stick to the bottom of the crockpot, wash it with warm water with drops of dishwashing solution. Set aside before drying and storing.

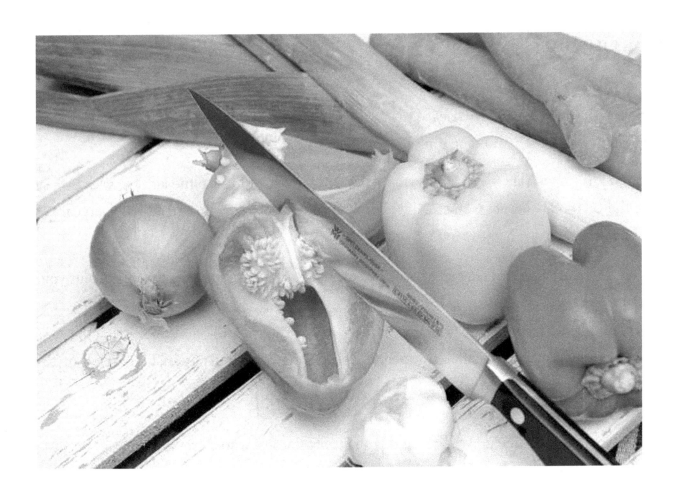

Conclusion

Living with Chronic Kidney Disease (CKD) doesn't mean that your life is about to end. You can still live long without being unduly affected by the condition.

Though it is impossible to amend the damage that is already done to the kidney, with proper care the CKD may not get worse. Even if your condition is mild, you must take good care of yourself. You can do so in the following ways:

- Take your medicine as prescribed, even if you are not feeling unwell, consult your doctor regularly.
- Have a healthy diet, it can help improve your general wellbeing and curtail the risks of developing further complications. A balanced diet may include some of the following:
- Eating plenty of fruits and vegetables.
- Meals that include starchy foods such as potatoes, whole grain bread, rice or pasta
- Dairy or dairy alternatives
- Low level of saturated fat, salt and sugar
- Engage in physical exercise regularly
- Avoid smoking
- Limit alcohol consumptions
- Be vaccinated - for disease
- Prevention.

Renal Diet Cookbook

Healthy Recipes with Low Sodium, Potassium and Phosphorus with a Precise Meal Prep Recipes Guide

SUSAN SIMON

Introduction

Managing chronic kidney disease (CKD) requires lifestyle adjustments, but it might help to know you're not alone. Over 31 million people in the United States are diagnosed with some malfunction of their kidneys or are battling kidney disease. As a registered dietitian (RD) with extensive experience assisting patients in taking control over their kidney disease, I have helped patients not only manage the physical symptoms associated with this disease but also cope with the emotional toll that this life change can take. Without knowing what the future holds, uncertainty, fear, depression, and anxiety can be common. It may even feel like dialysis is inevitable, and you may be asking yourself if it is worth the time or effort to try and manage this stage of the disease, or if it's even possible to delay the progression. As an expert in this field, I can assure you it is not just possible; it's yours to achieve—only 1 in 50 diagnosed with CKD end up on dialysis. So together, with the right tools, we can work to delay and ultimately prevent end-stage renal disease and dialysis. Success is earned through diet modifications and lifestyle changes. Using simple, manageable strategies, I have watched firsthand as my patients empowered themselves with knowledge. They have gone on to lead full, productive, and happy lives, continuing to work, play, and enjoy spending time with their loved ones— just the way it should be!

Only 1 in 50 diagnosed with CKD end up on dialysis

Diet is a vital part of treatment for CKD, and it can help immensely in slowing the progression of the disease. Some ingredients help the kidneys function, while others make the kidneys work harder. Also, targeting factors like salt and carbohydrate intake are important to reduce the risk of hypertension, diabetes, and other diseases that can result from kidney failure.

As an RD, I have years of firsthand experience treating patients at all stages of CKD. In this third book of my series, I want to give you, as a newly diagnosed individual, a better idea of how to manage these critical first stages with proper nutrition and recipes tailored to your unique condition. You may feel like you're in uncharted territory, and navigating your new dietary requirements can be challenging. At first, all of the new food dos and don'ts can be confusing, even frustrating, to you and your family. On top of that, it is common to be dealing with other health issues, such as hypertension or diabetes, which can add to the food restrictions.

It describes exactly what you can eat and what you should try to avoid, and features unique meal plans that can be tailored to your needs and likes. It will also provide you with specific diet information, such as the types of fruit with lower potassium, or the dairy choice with lower phosphorus, so you'll understand the best options when you prepare meals and snacks.

In this time of change and uncertainty, the knowledge you gain from these pages will give you the power to take your life into your hands and make changes to benefit you in the short and long term. I hope to educate and inspire you with new, easy ways to change the trajectory of your health. Adopting a kidney-friendly lifestyle can be challenging at first, but following these recipes will reduce the anxiety associated with selecting smart food options for your everyday life. And lest you worry that your new diet is restrictive or unsustainable, I want to assure you that these recipes are both easy and delicious, and they will give you a realistic, satisfying way to make this lifestyle change. In doing so, it will help take the stress of meal planning out of the equation and help you focus on the truly important things in life.

Chapeter 1: Introduction to Renal Diet

Since the Renal Diet is generally a Low Sodium, Low Phosphorus program, there are certain health benefits that you will enjoy from this diet. (Apart from improving your kidney health). Some of the crucial ones are as follows:

- It helps to lower blood pressure
- It helps to lower your LDL cholesterol
- It helps to lower your risk of having a heart attack
- It helps to prevent heart failure
- It decreases the possibility of having a stroke
- It helps to protect your vision
- It helps to improve your memory
- It helps to lower the possibility of dementia
- It helps to build stronger bones

Among others.

What Are the Symptoms of Chronic Kidney Disease?

CKD of Chronic Kidney diseases tends to eventually get worse as time passes. The unfortunate thing, though, is that the symptoms don't appear before the kidneys are damaged to a great extent.

During the later stages of CKD, though, as you reach almost complete kidney failure levels, you might start noticing various symptoms caused by toxin build-up in your body.

Some of the common symptoms include:

- Trouble when trying to sleep

- Breathing issues
- Abnormal urination
- Loss of appetite
- Constant feeling of nausea and vomit
- Body cramps all over
- Itching sensation all over

On the other hand, if your kidney suddenly stops working completely for some reason, you might experience more intense symptoms such as:

- Vomiting
- Rash all over
- Sudden nosebleeds
- Intense Diarrhea
- Intense Fever
- Abdominal Pain
- Back Pain

Having any one of the above-mentioned symptoms might be a sign that you might have a serious issue with your kidney. Instead of waiting, it's always best advised to consult with your physician as soon as possible.

Kidney Failure Treatment

If you are unfortunate enough to experience kidney failure, then you have two options.

You can look for a donor who might be able to donate one of their kidneys, or you may want to opt for dialysis.

Dialysis is an expensive and recurring process that you will need to do over and over again, depending on the condition of your kidneys.

Transplant, on the other hand, is mostly a one-time major expense, given that you can find a perfect match.

But regardless of the path you choose, there are thousands of people who have led a healthy and normal life, even with dialysis/kidney transplant. So, even if you are a victim, don't lose all your hopes just yet.

Let me talk a little bit about dialysis.

Dialysis is a process that helps to get rid of toxin and extra fluid build-up in your body through artificial means. However, an external machine won't be able to do everything that your kidney can do, so even with dialysis; you might face some complications in the long run.

That being said, there are two types of dialysis.

Peritoneal Dialysis

This form of treatment tries to cleanse your blood by utilizing the lining of your abdominal area and cleansing solution known as "Dialysate." The best part about this dialysis is that it can easily be done at home, as long as you have a clean and private area.

Hemodialysis

This particular treatment is also known as "Hemo" and is the most common one for kidney failures. This form of dialysis utilizes a machine to filter and clean out your blood. It is recommended that you do this at a hospital; however, if you have the budget, then it is possible to do it at home, as well.

After dialysis is the kidney transplant.

Kidney Transplant

A kidney transplant, as the name implies, is essentially surgery that gives you a healthy kidney from a donor's body. It is possible to have a kidney donated from a live body or a donor who has already died but has donated their kidney for a good cause. As mentioned above, if you can get a healthy kidney, then it is possible to lead a completely normal life.

And lastly, you can try medical management.

Medical Management

If you have budget issues or j want to avoid dialysis or transplant altogether, then there are some medical solutions that you might look into to reduce the symptoms of kidney failure.

They won't completely reverse the effects, but they might let you stay healthy until your kidneys are unable to function anymore.

If you opt for medical management, then the first thing to do is consult with your physician, as they will be able to point you in the right direction.

They will create a care plan for you that will guide you on what you should do and what you should not do. Make sure to always keep a copy of the plan wherever you go and discuss the terms with your loved ones as well.

It should be noted that most individuals who tend to go for medical management opt for hospice care.

The primary aim of hospice care is to try and decrease your pain and improve the quality of your final days before you die.

In medical management, you can expect a hospice to:

- Help you by providing you with a nursing home
- Help your family and friends to support you
- Try to improve the quality of your life as much as possible
- Try to provide medications and care to help you manage your symptoms

But keep in mind that regardless of which path you take, always discuss everything with your doctor.

Learning to Deal with Kidney Failure

Learning that you are suffering from kidney failure might be a difficult thing to cope with. No matter how long you have been preparing for the inevitable, this is something that will come as a shock to you.

But, as mentioned earlier, just because you have started dialysis, doesn't mean that everything that you hold dear has to come to an end!

It might be a little bit difficult at first to get yourself oriented to a new routine, but once you get into the groove, you'll start feeling much better.

Your nurses, loved ones, doctors, and co-workers will all be there to support you.

To make things easier, though, let me break down the individual types of problems that you might face and how you can deal with them.

Stress During Kidney Failure

When you are suffering from kidney failure, it's normal to be stressed out all the time. This might lead you to skip meals or even forgetting your medication, which might affect your health even more.

But you need to understand that life is full of hurdles and setbacks, and you really can't let them hold you back.

In that light, here are six tips to help you keep your stress under control:

- Make sure to take some time to just relax and unwind. Try to practice deep breathing, visualization, meditation or even muscle relaxation. All of these will help you to stay calm and keep your body healthy.
- Make sure to involve yourself in regular exercise. Take a hike, ride a bicycle or just simply take a jog. They all help. And if those aren't your thing, then you can always go for something more soothing, like tai chi or yoga.
- When you are feeling too stressed, try to call up a friend or a beloved family member and talk to them. And if that's not helping, you can always take help from a psychiatrist/counselor.
- Try to accept the things that are not under your control, and you can't change. Trying to enforce a change on something that is not within your reach will only

make things worse for you. Better advice is to look for better ways of handling the situation instead of trying to change it.

- Don't put too much pressure on yourself, try to be good to yourself and don't expect much. You are a human being, after all, right? You can make mistakes, so accept that. Just try your best.

- And lastly, always try to maintain a positive attitude. Even when things go completely wrong, try to see the good instead of the bad and focus on that. Try to find things in all phases of your life that make you happy and that you appreciate, such as your friends, work, health and family, for example. You have no idea how much help a simple change of perspective can bring.

And on the topic of working out.

Exercise

Apart from the special diet, such as the Renal Diet, physical activity is another way through which you can improve the quality of your life.

This might be a little bit tough to do if you are alone, but it is very much possible. However, you should keep in mind that working out alone won't help you; you must work out and follow a well-balanced, healthy diet.

Both of these combined will go to great lengths to help you lose weight and control your disease.

A study has shown that people who try to complete 10,1000 steps per day and work out for about 2½ hours every week, while cutting down 500-800 calories per day and following a proper diet routine, have a 50% chance of reducing blood sugar to normal levels, which will further help you to stay healthy.

Common forms of exercise include:

- Stair climbing
- Tai Chi

- Stretching
- Yoga
- Cycling
- Walking
- Swimming

And so on.

To perform these normal workouts, you don't have to join a gym or even buy any sort of expensive equipment! You can simply take a walk around your streets, do yoga at home, and so on.

Just make sure to consult with your doctor to find out which exercise is suitable for you and adjust them to your dialysis routine.

Anxiety and Depression

These two are possibly the most prominent issues that you are going to face. A feeling of depression might last for a long period if left unattended. Anxiety might come at the same time, but it won't last for long.

Either way, mood swings will occur that will suddenly make you sad.

However, you should know that it is completely normal to feel anxious or sad when you're going through such a huge change in life. This is even more prominent if you start taking dialysis, as it will require you to completely change your daily routine and follow a different type of diet.

During this adjusting phase, you'll feel many emotions, such as anger, fear, sadness, etc.

To summarize:

The symptoms of depression are:

- Loss of interest
- Loss of any appetite

- Sleeping problems

On the other hand, symptoms of anxiety are:

- Constant sweating
- Quick breathing
- Inconsistent heartbeat
- Constant troubling thoughts

Regardless, the main thing to know is that you are not alone in this fight. Thousands of people have and are going through the same experience. Many people often feel left alone and lose the will to fight, but it doesn't have to be the same for you.

Help is always available! Try sharing with your family members, join support groups, talk to a social worker, etc.

It doesn't matter what your situation is; if you just reach out to the right person, then you will always find the help and support that you need.

Is it Possible to Work During Dialysis?

Some people often think that you have to stop working or retire from your job the moment you start taking dialysis. But that's not necessarily true.

It is very much possible to keep working even after you start dialysis. It is recommended that you try to continue working to stay happier and healthier.

If your company provides health insurance, then you can even keep enjoying the benefits of insurance while you work. It will help you bear the costs of your dialysis as well.

There are some types of dialysis that provide more flexible treatment options, allowing you to have more time during the day for your job.

Nocturnal (Night-Time) dialysis, either at home or hospital, is perfect for these.

However, if you do start working during your dialysis, you should understand your limits. While you are working, it is possible that you might feel bit weak or tired.

If you are following peritoneal dialysis, then you are going to need a clean place to do all your exchanges.

Alternatively, if you are on Hemo, then it is strictly prohibited for you to lift heavy objects or put excess pressure on your vascular access arm.

Depending on your dialysis type, you must talk to your social worker/doctor to adjust your dialysis routine and talk to your employer to reach an agreement.

Worst case scenario, if you are unable to work, you still have some options! Various federal and private programs will help you to have a stable income while keeping your insurance for your dialysis program.

Talk to your social worker to apply for these facilities.

Chapeter 2: Benefits of Renal Diet

One of the most effective ways to prevent kidney disease is with proper diet.

It's also important to know that those who are at risk of this disease or have already been diagnosed with this condition can help alleviate symptoms and slow down the progression of the disease with a diet called the renal diet.

As you know, the wastes in the blood come from the foods and drinks that you consume.

When your kidneys are not functioning properly, they are unable to remove these wastes efficiently.

Wastes that remain in the blood can negatively affect your overall health.

Following a renal diet can help bolster the functioning of the kidney, reduce damage to the kidneys and prevent kidney failure.

A renal diet is a type of diet that involves consumption of foods and drinks that are low in potassium, sodium and phosphorus.

It also puts focus on the consumption of high-quality protein as well as limiting too much intake of fluids and calcium.

Since each person's body is different, it's important to come up with a specific diet formulated by a dietician to make sure that the diet is tailored to the needs of the patient.

Some of the substances that you have to check and monitor for proper renal diet include:

The Benefits of Renal Diet

A renal diet minimizes intake of sodium, potassium and phosphorus.

Excessive sodium is harmful to people who have been diagnosed with kidney disease as this causes fluid buildup, making it hard for the kidneys to eliminate sodium and fluid.

Improper functioning of the kidneys can also mean difficulty in removing excess potassium.

When there is too much potassium in the body, this can lead to a condition called hyperkalemia, which can also cause problems with the heart and blood vessels.

Kidneys that are not working efficiently find it difficult to remove excess phosphorus.

High levels of phosphorus excrete calcium from the bones causing them to weaken. This also causes elevation of calcium deposits in the eyes, heart, lungs, and blood vessels.

Chapter 3: What You Can Eat And What You Can Avoid In Renal Diet

A renal diet focuses on foods that are natural and nutritious, but at the same time, are low in sodium, potassium and phosphorus.

Foods to eat:

Cauliflower - 1 cup contains 19 mg sodium, 176 potassium, 40 mg phosphorus

Blueberries - 1 cup contains 1.5 mg sodium, 114 potassium, 18 mg phosphorus

Sea Bass - 3 ounces contain 74 mg sodium, 279 potassium, 211 mg phosphorus

Grapes - 1/2 cup contains 1.5 mg sodium, 144 potassium, 15 mg phosphorus

Egg Whites - 2 egg whites contain 110 mg sodium, 108 potassium, 10 mg phosphorus

Garlic - 3 cloves contain 1.5 mg sodium, 36 potassium, 14 mg phosphorus

Buckwheat - ½ cup contains 3.5 mg sodium, 74 potassium, 59 mg phosphorus

Olive Oil - 1 ounce 0.6 mg sodium, 0.3 potassium, 0 mg phosphorus

Bulgur - ½ cup contains 4.5 mg sodium, 62 potassium, 36 mg phosphorus

Cabbage - 1 cup contains 13 mg sodium, 119 potassium, 18 mg phosphorus

Skinless chicken - 3 ounces contain 63 mg sodium, 216 potassium, 192 mg phosphorus

Bell peppers - 1 piece contains 3 mg sodium, 156 potassium, 19 mg phosphorus

Onion - 1 piece contains 3 mg sodium, 102 potassium, 20 mg phosphorus

Arugula - 1 cup contains 6 mg sodium, 74 potassium, 10 mg phosphorus

Macadamia nuts - 1 ounce contains 1.4 mg sodium, 103 potassium, 53 mg phosphorus

Radish - ½ cup contains 23 mg sodium, 135 potassium, 12 mg phosphorus

Turnips - ½ cup contains 12.5 mg sodium, 138 potassium, 20 mg phosphorus

Pineapple - 1 cup contains 2 mg sodium, 180 potassium, 13 mg phosphorus

Cranberries – 1 cup contains 2 mg sodium, 85 potassium, 13 mg phosphorus

Mushrooms – 1 cup contains 6 mg sodium, 170 potassium, 42 mg phosphorus

Foods to Avoid

These foods are known to have high levels of potassium, sodium or phosphorus:

Soda – Soda is believed to contain up to 100 mg of additive phosphorus per 200 ml.

Avocados - 1 cup contains up to 727 mg of potassium.

Canned foods – Canned foods contain high amounts of sodium so make sure that you avoid using these, or at least, opt for low-sodium versions.

Whole wheat bread – 1 ounce of bread contains 57 mg phosphorus and 69 mg potassium, which is higher compared to white bread.

Brown rice – 1 cup of brown rice contains 154 mg potassium while 1 cup of white rice only has 54 mg potassium.

Bananas – 1 banana contains 422 mg of potassium.

Dairy – Dairy products are high in potassium, phosphorus and calcium. You can still consume dairy products but you have to limit it. Use dairy milk alternatives like almond milk and coconut milk.

Processed Meats – Processed meats are not advisable to people with kidney problems because of their high content of additives and preservatives.

Pickled and cured foods – These are made using large amounts of salt.

Apricots – 1 cup contains 427 mg potassium.

Potatoes and sweet potatoes – 1 potato contain 610 mg potassium. You can double boil potatoes and sweet potatoes to reduce potassium by 50 percent.

Tomatoes – 1 cup tomato sauce contains up to 900 mg potassium.

Instant meals – Instant meals are known for extremely high amounts of sodium.

Spinach – Spinach contains up to 290 mg potassium per cup. Cooking helps reduce the amount of potassium.

Raisins, prunes and dates – Dried fruits have concentrated nutrients including potassium. 1 cup prunes contain up to 1,274 mg potassium.

Chips – Chips are known to have high amounts of sodium.

Since the Renal Diet is generally a Low Sodium, Low Phosphorus program, there are certain health benefits that you will enjoy from this diet. (Apart from improving your kidney health). Some of the crucial ones are as follows:

- It helps to lower blood pressure
- It helps to lower your LDL cholesterol
- It helps to lower your risk of having a heart attack
- It helps to prevent heart failure
- It decreases the possibility of having a stroke
- It helps to protect your vision
- It helps to improve your memory
- It helps to lower the possibility of dementia
- It helps to build stronger bones

Chapter 4: Breakfast Recipes

1. Chicken Egg Rolls

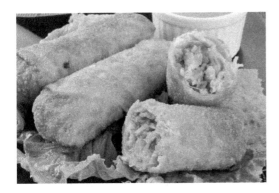

Preparation time: 10 minutes

Cooking time: 12 minutes

Servings: 14

Ingredients:

1 lb. cooked chicken, diced

1/2 lb. bean sprouts

1/2 lb. cabbage, shredded

1 cup onion, chopped

2 tablespoons olive oil

1 tablespoon low sodium soy sauce

1 garlic clove, minced

20 egg roll wrappers

Oil for frying

Directions:

Add everything to a suitable bowl except for the roll wrappers.

Mix these ingredients well to prepare the filling then marinate for 30 minutes.

Place the roll wrappers on the working surface and divide the prepared filling on them.

Fold the roll wrappers as per the package instructions and keep them aside.

Add oil to a deep wok and heat it to 350 degrees F.

Deep the egg rolls until golden brown on all sides.

Transfer the egg rolls to a plate lined with a paper towel to absorb all the excess oil.

Serve warm.

Nutrition:

Calories 212

Total Fat 3.8g

Saturated Fat 0.7g

Cholesterol 29mg

Sodium 329mg

Carbohydrate 29g

Dietary Fiber 1.4g

Sugars 0.9g

Protein 14.9g

Calcium 37mg

Phosphorous 361 mg

Potassium 171mg

2. Pork Bread Casserole

Preparation time: 20 minutes

Cooking time: 55 minutes

Servings: 8

Ingredients:

2 tablespoons butter

1 lb. pork sausage

1 yellow onion, chopped

18 slices white bread, cut into cubes

2 ½ cups sharp Cheddar cheese, grated

1/2 cup fresh parsley, chopped

6 large eggs

2 cups half-and-half cream

1 teaspoon garlic powder

1/4 teaspoon black pepper

Directions:

Switch on your gas oven and preheat it at 325 degrees F.

Layer a 9x9 inches casserole dish with bread cubes.

Set a suitable-sized skillet over medium-high heat then crumb the sausage in it.

Cook the sausage until golden brown, then keep it aside.

Blend the eggs with the remaining ingredients in a blender until smooth.

Stir in the sausage and spread this mixture over the bread pieces.

Bake the bread casserole for 55 minutes approximately in the preheated oven.

Slice and serve.

Enjoy.

Nutrition:

Calories 366

Total Fat 26.4g

Saturated Fat 15.1g

Cholesterol 208mg Sodium 436mg

Carbohydrate 15.2g

Dietary Fiber 0.9g Sugars 2.1g

Protein 17.5g Calcium 378mg

Phosphorous 501 mg

Potassium 231mg

3. Salmon Bagel Toast

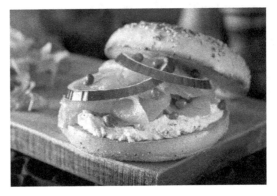

Preparation time: 10 minutes

Cooking time: 5 minutes

Servings: 2

Ingredients:

1 plain bagel, cut in half

2 tablespoons cream cheese

1/3 cup English cucumber, thinly sliced

3 oz. smoked salmon, sliced

3 rings red onion

1/2 teaspoon capers, drained

Directions:

Toast each half of the bagel in a skillet until golden brown.

Cover one of the toasted halves with cream cheese.

Set the cucumber, salmon, and capers on top of each bagel half.

Enjoy.

Nutrition: Calories 223

Total Fat 6.2g Saturated Fat 2.8g

Cholesterol 21mg Sodium 1137mg

Carbohydrate 27.5g Dietary Fiber 1.3g

Sugars 3g

Protein 13.9g

Calcium 62mg

Phosphorous 79mg

Potassium 151mg

4. Cinnamon Toast Strata

Preparation time: 10 minutes

Cooking time: 50 minutes

Servings: 12

Ingredients:

1 lb. loaf cinnamon raisin bread, cubed

8 oz. package cream cheese, diced

1 cup apples, peeled and diced

8 eggs

2 1/2 cups half-and-half cream

6 tablespoons butter, melted

1/4 cup maple syrup

Directions:

Layer a 9x13 inch baking dish with cooking spray.

Place ½ of the bread cubes in the greased baking dish.

Cover the bread cubes with cream cheese, apples, and the other half of the bread.

Beat the eggs with the melted butter and maple syrup in a bowl.

Pour this egg-butter mixture over the bread layer then refrigerate for 2 hours.

Bake this bread-egg casserole for 50 minutes at 325 degrees F.

Slice and garnish with pancake syrup.

Enjoy.

Nutrition:

Calories 276

Total Fat 21.4g

Saturated Fat 12.4g

Cholesterol 165mg

Sodium 206mg

Carbohydrate 14.5g

Dietary Fiber 0.6g

Sugars 7.4g

Protein 7.5g

Calcium 90mg

Phosphorous 263 mg

Potassium 162mg

5. Cottage Cheese Pancakes

Preparation time: 10 minutes

Cooking time: 10 minutes

Servings: 4

Ingredients: 1 cup cottage cheese

1/3 cup all-purpose flour

2 tablespoons vegetable oil

3 eggs, lightly beaten

Directions: Begin by beating the eggs in a suitable bowl then stir in the cottage cheese. Once it is well mixed, stir in the flour. Pour a teaspoon of vegetable oil in a non-stick griddle and heat it. Add ¼ cup of the batter in the griddle and cook for 2 minutes per side until brown. Cook more of the pancakes using the remaining batter. Serve.

Nutrition: Calories 196   Total Fat 11.3g Saturated Fat 3.1g Cholesterol 127mg

Sodium 276mg Carbohydrate 10.3g

Dietary Fiber 0.3g Sugars 0.5g

Protein 13g   Calcium 58mg

Phosphorous 187 mg Potassium 110mg

6. Asparagus Bacon Hash

Preparation time: 10 minutes

Cooking time: 27 minutes

Servings: 4

Ingredients:

6 slices bacon, diced

1/2 onion, chopped

2 cloves garlic, sliced

2 lb. asparagus, trimmed and chopped

Black pepper, to taste

2 tablespoons Parmesan, grated

4 large eggs

1/4 teaspoon red pepper flakes

Directions:

Add the asparagus and a tablespoon of water to a microwave-proof bowl.

Cover the veggies and microwave them for 5 minutes until tender.

Set a suitable non-stick skillet over moderate heat and layer it with cooking spray.

Stir in the onion and sauté for 7 minutes, then toss in the garlic.

Stir for 1 minute, then toss in the asparagus, eggs, and red pepper flakes.

Reduce the heat to low and cover the vegetables in the pan. Top the eggs with Parmesan cheese.

Cook for approximately 15 minutes, then slice to serve.

Nutrition:

Calories 290

Total Fat 17.9g

Saturated Fat 6.1g

Cholesterol 220mg

Sodium 256mg

Carbohydrate 11.6g

Dietary Fiber 5.1g

Sugars 5.3g

Protein 23.2g

Calcium 121mg

Phosphorous 247mg

Potassium 715mg

7. Cheese Spaghetti Frittata

Preparation time: 10 minutes

Cooking time: 10 minutes

Servings: 6

Ingredients:

4 cups whole-wheat spaghetti, cooked

4 teaspoons olive oil

3 medium onions, chopped

4 large eggs

½ cup milk

⅓ cup Parmesan cheese, grated

2 tablespoons fresh parsley, chopped

2 tablespoons fresh basil, chopped

½ teaspoon black pepper

1 tomato, diced

Directions:

Set a suitable non-stick skillet over moderate heat and add in the olive oil.

Place the spaghetti in the skillet and cook by stirring for 2 minutes on moderate heat.

Whisk the eggs with milk, parsley, and black pepper in a bowl.

Pour this milky egg mixture over the spaghetti and top it all with basil, cheese, and tomato.

Cover the spaghetti frittata again with a lid and cook for approximately 8 minutes on low heat.

Slice and serve.

Nutrition:

Calories 230

Total Fat 7.8g

Saturated Fat 2g

Cholesterol 127mg

Sodium 77mg

Carbohydrate 31.9g

Dietary Fiber 5.6g

Sugars 4.5g

Protein 11.1g

Calcium 88mg

Phosphorous 368 mg

Potassium 214mg

8. Pineapple Bread

Preparation time: 20 minutes

Cooking time: 1 hour

Servings: 10

Ingredients:

1/3 cup Swerve

1/3 cup butter, unsalted

2 eggs

2 cups flour

3 teaspoons baking powder

1 cup pineapple, undrained

6 cherries, chopped

Directions:

Whisk the Swerve with the butter in a mixer until fluffy.

Stir in the eggs, then beat again.

Add the baking powder and flour, then mix well until smooth.

Fold in the cherries and pineapple.

Spread this cherry-pineapple batter in a 9x5 inch baking pan.

Bake the pineapple batter for 1 hour at 350 degrees F.

Slice the bread and serve.

Nutrition:

Calories 197

Total Fat 7.2g

Saturated Fat 1.3g

Cholesterol 33mg

Sodium 85mg

Carbohydrate 18.3g

Dietary Fiber 1.1g

Sugars 3 g

Protein 4g

Calcium 79mg

Phosphorous 316mg

Potassium 227mg

9. Parmesan Zucchini Frittata

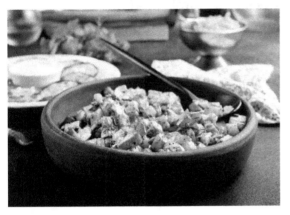

Preparation time: 10 minutes

Cooking time: 35 minutes

Servings: 6

Ingredients:

1 tablespoon olive oil

1 cup yellow onion, sliced

3 cups zucchini, chopped

½ cup Parmesan cheese, grated

8 large eggs

½ teaspoon black pepper

⅛ teaspoon paprika

3 tablespoons parsley, chopped

Directions:

Toss the zucchinis with the onion, parsley, and all other ingredients in a large bowl.

Pour this zucchini-garlic mixture in an 11x7 inches pan and spread it evenly.

Bake the zucchini casserole for approximately 35 minutes at 350 degrees F.

Cut in slices and serve.

Nutrition:

Calories 142

Total Fat 9.7g

Saturated Fat 2.8g

Cholesterol 250mg

Sodium 123mg

Carbohydrate 4.7g

Dietary Fiber 1.3g

Sugars 2.4g

Protein 10.2g

Calcium 73mg

Phosphorous 375mg

Potassium 286mg

10. Texas Toast Casserole

Preparation time: 10 minutes

Cooking time: 30 minutes

Servings: 10

Ingredients:

1/2 cup butter, melted

1 cup brown Swerve

1 lb. Texas Toast bread, sliced

4 large eggs

1 1/2 cup milk

1 tablespoon vanilla extract

2 tablespoons Swerve

2 teaspoons cinnamon

Maple syrup for serving

Directions:

Layer a 9x13 inches baking pan with cooking spray.

Spread the bread slices at the bottom of the prepared pan.

Whisk the eggs with the remaining ingredients in a mixer.

Pour this mixture over the bread slices evenly.

Bake the bread for 30 minutes at 350 degrees F in a preheated oven.

Serve.

Nutrition:

Calories 332

Total Fat 13.7g

Saturated Fat 6.9g

Cholesterol 102mg

Sodium 350mg

Carbohydrate 22.6g

Dietary Fiber 2g

Sugars 6g

Protein 7.4g

Calcium 143mg

Phosphorous 186mg

Potassium 74mg

11. Apple Cinnamon Rings

Preparation time: 10 minutes

Cooking time: 20 minutes

Servings: 6

Ingredients:

4 large apples, cut in rings

1 cup flour

¼ teaspoon baking powder

1 teaspoon stevia

¼ teaspoon cinnamon

1 large egg, beaten

1 cup milk

Vegetable oil, for frying

Cinnamon Topping:

⅓ cup of brown Swerve

2 teaspoons cinnamon

Directions:

Begin by mixing the flour with the baking powder, cinnamon, and stevia in a bowl.

Whisk the egg with the milk in a bowl.

Stir in the dry flour mixture and mix well until it makes a smooth batter.

Pour oil into a wok to deep fry the rings and heat it to 375 degrees F.

First, dip the apple in the flour batter and deep fry until golden brown.

Transfer the apple rings on a tray lined with a paper towel.

Drizzle the cinnamon and Swerve topping over the slices.

Serve fresh in the morning.

Nutrition:

Calories 166

Total Fat 1.7g

Saturated Fat 0.5g

Cholesterol 33mg

Sodium 55mg

Carbohydrate 13.1g

Dietary Fiber 1.9g Sugars 6.9g

Protein 4.7g Calcium 65mg

Phosphorous 241mg

Potassium 197mg

12.Zucchini Bread

Preparation time: 20 minutes

Cooking time: 1 hour

Servings: 16

Ingredients:

3 eggs

1 1/2 cups Swerve

1 cup apple sauce

2 cups zucchini, shredded

1 teaspoon vanilla

2 cups flour

1/4 teaspoon baking powder

1 teaspoon baking soda

1 teaspoon cinnamon

1/2 teaspoon ginger

1 cup unsalted nuts, chopped

Directions:

Thoroughly whisk the eggs with the zucchini, apple sauce, and the rest of the ingredients in a bowl.

Once mixed evenly, spread the mixture in a loaf pan.

Bake it for 1 hour at 375 degrees F in a preheated oven.

Slice and serve.

Nutrition: Calories 200

Total Fat 5.4g Saturated Fat 0.9g

Cholesterol 31mg Sodium 94mg

Carbohydrate 26.9g Dietary Fiber 1.6g

Sugars 16.3g Protein 4.4g

Calcium 20mg Phosphorous 212mg

Potassium 137mg

13. Garlic Mayo Bread

Preparation time: 10 minutes

Cooking time: 5 minutes

Servings: 16

Ingredients:

3 tablespoons vegetable oil

4 cloves garlic, minced

2 teaspoons paprika

Dash cayenne pepper

1 teaspoon lemon juice

2 tablespoons Parmesan cheese, grated

3/4 cup mayonnaise

1 loaf (1 lb.) French bread, sliced

1 teaspoon Italian herbs

Directions:

Mix the garlic with the oil in a small bowl and leave it overnight.

Discard the garlic from the bowl and keep the garlic-infused oil.

Mix the garlic-oil with cayenne, paprika, lemon juice, mayonnaise, and Parmesan.

Place the bread slices in a baking tray lined with parchment paper.

Top these slices with the mayonnaise mixture and drizzle the Italian herbs on top.

Broil these slices for 5 minutes until golden brown.

Serve warm.

Nutrition:

Calories 217

Total Fat 7.9g

Saturated Fat 1.8g

Cholesterol 5mg

Sodium 423mg

Carbohydrate 30.3g

Dietary Fiber 1.3g

Sugars 2g Protein 7g

Calcium 56mg Phosphorous 347mg

Potassium 72mg

14. Strawberry Topped Waffles

Preparation time: 15 minutes

Cooking time: 20 minutes

Servings: 5

Ingredients:

1 cup flour

1/4 cup Swerve

1 ¾ teaspoons baking powder

1 egg, separated

¾ cup milk

½ cup butter, melted

½ teaspoon vanilla extract

Fresh strawberries, sliced

Directions:

Prepare and preheat your waffle pan following the instructions of the machine. Begin by mixing the flour with Swerve and baking soda in a bowl.

Separate the egg yolks from the egg whites, keeping them in two separate bowls. Add the milk and vanilla extract to the egg yolks. Stir the melted butter and mix well until smooth. Now beat the egg whites with an electric beater until foamy and fluffy. Fold this fluffy composition in the egg yolk mixture. Mix it gently until smooth, then add in the flour mixture. Stir again to make a smooth mixture. Pour a half cup of the waffle batter in a preheated pan and cook until the waffle is done. Cook more waffles with the remaining batter.

Serve fresh with strawberries on top.

Nutrition: Calories 342 Total Fat 20.5g

Saturated Fat 12.5g Cholesterol 88mg

Sodium 156mg Carbohydrate 21g

Dietary Fiber 0.7g

Sugars 3.5g

Protein 4.8g

Calcium 107mg

Phosphorous 126mg

Potassium 233mg

15. Mixed Pepper Mushroom Omelet

Preparation time: 10 minutes

Cooking time: 10 minutes

Servings: 2

Ingredients:

1/4 cup green onions, chopped

1/4 cup fresh mushrooms, sliced

1/4 cup green pepper, chopped

2 tablespoons butter, divided

5 eggs

1/4 teaspoon pepper

1/4 cup Cheddar cheese, shredded

1/4 cup Monterey Jack cheese, shredded

Directions:

Begin by sautéing all the vegetables with the butter in a pan until crispy.

Whisk the eggs and black pepper until foamy and fluffy.

Spread this egg mixture over the vegetables in the pan and cover with a lid.

Cook for about 2 minutes, then flip the omelet with a spatula.

Drizzle the cheese on top and cover the lid for 2 more minutes.

Slice and serve.

Nutrition:

Calories 378

Total Fat 31.5g

Saturated Fat 16.4g

Cholesterol 467mg

Sodium 402mg

Carbohydrate 3.1g

Dietary Fiber 0.7g

Sugars 1.7g

Protein 21.6g

Calcium 280mg

Phosphorous 412mg

Potassium 262mg

16.Mozzarella Cheese Omelette

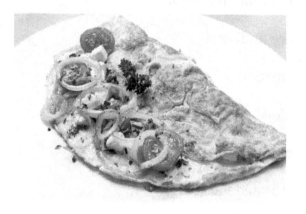

Preparation Time: 10 minutes

Cooking Time: 5 minutes

Servings: 1

Ingredients:

4 eggs, beaten

1/4 cup mozzarella cheese, shredded

4 tomato slices

1/4 tsp Italian seasoning

1/4 tsp dried oregano

Pepper

Salt

Directions:

In a small bowl, whisk eggs with salt.

Spray pan with cooking spray and heat over medium heat.

Pour egg mixture into the pan and cook over medium heat.

Once eggs are set then sprinkle oregano and Italian seasoning on top.

Arrange tomato slices on top of the omelet and sprinkle with shredded cheese.

Cook omelet for 1 minute.

Serve and enjoy.

Nutrition: Calories 285 Fat 19 g Carbohydrates 4 g Sugar 3 g Protein 25 g Cholesterol 655 mg

17. Sun-Dried Tomato Frittata

Preparation Time: 10 minutes

Cooking Time: 20 minutes

Servings: 8

Ingredients: 1/2 tsp dried basil

12 eggs

1/4 cup parmesan cheese, grated

2 cups baby spinach, shredded

1/4 cup sun-dried tomatoes, sliced

Pepper - Salt

Directions: Preheat the oven to 425 F. In a large bowl, whisk eggs with pepper and salt. Add remaining ingredients and stir to combine. Spray oven-safe pan with cooking spray. Pour egg mixture into the pan and bake for 20 minutes.

Slice and serve.

Nutrition: Calories 115 Fat 7 g Carbohydrates 1 g Sugar 1 g Protein 10 g Cholesterol 250 mg

18. Italian Breakfast Frittata

Preparation Time: 10 minutes

Cooking Time: 45 minutes

Servings: 4

Ingredients:

2 cups egg whites

1/2 cup mozzarella cheese, shredded

1 cup cottage cheese, crumbled

1/4 cup fresh basil, sliced

1/2 cup roasted red peppers, sliced

Pepper

Salt

Directions:

Preheat the oven to 375 F.

Add all ingredients into the large bowl and whisk well to combine.

Pour frittata mixture into the baking dish and bake for 45 minutes. Slice and serve.

Nutrition: Calories 131 Fat 2 g Carbohydrates 5 g Sugar 2 g Protein 22 g Cholesterol 6 mg

19. Sausage Cheese Bake Omelette

Preparation Time: 10 minutes

Cooking Time: 45 minutes

Servings: 8

Ingredients: 16 eggs

2 cups cheddar cheese, shredded

1/2 cup salsa

1 lb ground sausage

1 1/2 cups coconut milk

Pepper - Salt

Directions: Preheat the oven to 350 F.

Add sausage in a pan and cook until browned. Drain excess fat.

In a large bowl, whisk eggs and milk. Stir in cheese, cooked sausage, and salsa.

Pour omelet mixture into the baking dish and bake for 45 minutes.

Serve and enjoy.

Nutrition: Calories   360   Fat   24   g Carbohydrates 4 g Sugar 3 g Protein 28 g Cholesterol 400 mg

20.   Greek Egg Scrambled

Preparation Time: 10 minutes

Cooking Time: 10 minutes

Servings: 2

Ingredients: 1/2 cup grape tomatoes, sliced   - 4 eggs

2 tbsp green onions, sliced

1 bell pepper, diced   - 1 tbsp olive oil

1/4 tsp dried oregano

1/2 tbsp capers

3 olives, sliced

Pepper - Salt

Directions: Heat oil in a pan over medium heat.   Add green onions and bell pepper and cook until pepper is softened.   Add tomatoes, capers, and olives and cook for 1 minute.   Add eggs and stir until eggs are cooked. Season with oregano, pepper, and salt. Serve and enjoy.

Nutrition: Calories   230   Fat   17   g Carbohydrates 8 g Sugar 5 g Protein 12 g Cholesterol 325 mg

21. Feta Mint Omelette

Preparation Time: 10 minutes

Cooking Time: 5 minutes

Servings: 1

Ingredients:

3 eggs

1/4 cup fresh mint, chopped

2 tbsp coconut milk

1/2 tsp olive oil

2 tbsp feta cheese, crumbled

Pepper

Salt

Directions:

In a bowl, whisk eggs with feta cheese, mint, milk, pepper, and salt.

Heat olive oil in a pan over low heat.

Pour egg mixture in the pan and cook until eggs are set. Flip omelet and cook for 2 minutes more. Serve and enjoy.

Nutrition: Calories 275 Fat 20 g Carbohydrates 4 g Sugar 2 g Protein 20 g Cholesterol 505 mg

22. Sausage Breakfast Casserole

Preparation Time: 10 minutes

Cooking Time: 50 minutes

Servings: 8

Ingredients: 1 lb. ground Italian sausage - 12 eggs

2 1/2 tomatoes, sliced

3 tbsp coconut flour 1/4 cup coconut milk 2 small zucchinis, shredded

Pepper   - Salt

Directions: Preheat the oven to 350 F. Spray casserole dish with cooking spray and set aside. Cook sausage in a pan until brown. Transfer sausage to a mixing bowl. Add coconut flour, milk, eggs, zucchini, pepper, and salt. Stir well. Add eggs and whisk to combine. Transfer bowl mixture into the casserole dish and top with tomato slices. Bake for 50 minutes. Serve and enjoy.

Nutrition: Calories 305 Fat 21.8 g Carbohydrates 6.3 g Sugar 3.3 g Protein 19.6 g Cholesterol 286 mg

23. Easy Turnip Puree

Preparation Time: 10 minutes

Cooking Time: 12 minutes

Servings: 4

Ingredients:

1 1/2 lbs. turnips, peeled and chopped

1 tsp dill

3 bacon slices, cooked and chopped

2 tbsp fresh chives, chopped

Directions:

Add turnip into the boiling water and cook for 12 minutes. Drain well and place in a food processor.

Add dill and process until smooth.

Transfer turnip puree into the bowl and top with bacon and chives.

Serve and enjoy.

Nutrition: Calories 127 Fat 6 g Carbohydrates 11.6 g Sugar 7 g Protein 6.8 g Cholesterol 16 mg

24. Spinach Bacon Breakfast Bake

Preparation Time: 10 minutes

Cooking Time: 45 minutes

Servings: 6

Ingredients: 3 cups baby spinach, chopped   1 tbsp olive oil   10 eggs

8 bacon slices, cooked and chopped

2 tomatoes, sliced

2 tbsp chives, chopped

Pepper - Salt

Directions: Preheat the oven to 350 F. Spray a baking dish with cooking spray and set aside.   Heat oil in a pan. Add spinach and cook until spinach wilted. In a mixing bowl, whisk eggs and salt. Add spinach and chives and stir well. Pour egg mixture into the baking dish.   Top with tomatoes and bacon and bake for 45 minutes. Serve and enjoy.

Nutrition: Calories 273 Fat 20.4 g Carbohydrates 3.1 g Sugar 1.7 g Protein 19.4 g Cholesterol 301 mg

25. Healthy Spinach Tomato Muffins

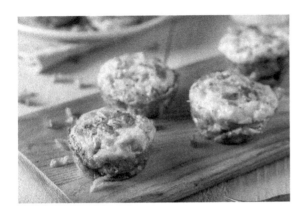

Preparation Time: 10 minutes

Cooking Time: 20 minutes

Servings: 12

Ingredients:

12 eggs

1/2 tsp Italian seasoning

1 cup tomatoes, chopped

4 tbsp water

1 cup fresh spinach, chopped

Pepper

Salt

Directions:

Preheat the oven to 350 F.

Spray a muffin tray with cooking spray and set aside.

In a mixing bowl, whisk eggs with water, Italian seasoning, pepper, and salt.

Add spinach and tomatoes and stir well.

Pour egg mixture into the prepared muffin tray and bake for 20 minutes.

Serve and enjoy.

Nutrition: Calories 67 Fat 4.5 g Carbohydrates 1 g Sugar 0.8 g Protein 5.7 g Cholesterol 164 mg

Chapter 5: Lunch Recipes

26.   Cauliflower Rice and Coconut

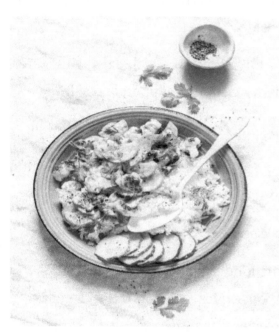

Serving: 4

Prep Time: 20 minutes

Cook Time: 20 minutes

Ingredients:

3 cups cauliflower, riced

2/3 cups full-fat coconut milk

1-2 teaspoons sriracha paste

¼- ½ teaspoon onion powder

Salt as needed

Fresh basil for garnish

Directions:

Take a pan and place it over medium-low heat

Add all of the ingredients and stir them until fully combined

Cook for about 5-10 minutes, making sure that the lid is on

Remove the lid and keep cooking until there's no excess liquid

Once the rice is soft and creamy, enjoy it!

Nutrition:

Calories: 95

Fat: 7g

Carbohydrates: 4g

Protein: 1g

Kale and Garlic Platter

Preparation Time: 5 minutes

Cooking Time: 10 minutes

Servings: 4

Ingredients:

1 bunch kale

2 tablespoons olive oil

4 garlic cloves, minced

Directions:

Carefully tear the kale into bite-sized portions, making sure to remove the stem

Discard the stems Take a large-sized pot and place it over medium heat Add olive oil and let the oil heat up Add garlic and stir for 2 minutes Add kale and cook for 5-10 minutes Serve!

Nutrition

Calories: 121

Fat: 8g Carbohydrates: 5g

Protein: 4g

27. Blistered Beans and Almond

Preparation Time: 10 minutes

Cooking Time: 20 minutes

Servings: 4

Ingredients: 1 pound fresh green beans, ends trimmed - 1 ½ tablespoon olive oil

¼ teaspoon salt - 1 ½ tablespoons fresh dill, minced - Juice of 1 lemon - Salt as needed

¼ cup crushed almonds

Directions: Preheat your oven to 400 °F Add in the green beans with your olive oil and also the salt Then spread them in one single layer on a large-sized sheet pan Roast for 10 minutes and stir nicely, then roast for another 8-10 minutes Remove it from the oven and keep stirring in the lemon juice alongside the dill Top it with crushed almonds, some flaky sea salt and serve

Nutrition: Calories: 347 Fat: 16g

Carbohydrates: 6g Protein: 45g

28. Cucumber Soup

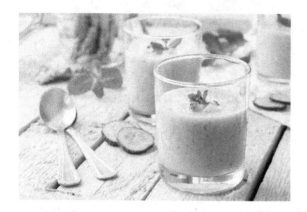

Preparation Time: 14 minutes

Cooking Time: Nil

Servings: 4

Ingredients:

2 tablespoons garlic, minced

4 cups English cucumbers, peeled and diced

½ cup onions, diced

1 tablespoon lemon juice

1 ½ cups vegetable broth

½ teaspoon salt

¼ teaspoon red pepper flakes

¼ cup parsley, diced

½ cup Greek yogurt, plain

Directions:

Add the listed ingredients to a blender and emulsify by blending them (except ½ cup of chopped cucumbers)

Blend until smooth

Divide the soup amongst 4 servings and top with extra cucumbers

Enjoy chilled!

Nutrition

Calories: 371

Fat: 36g

Carbohydrates: 8g

Protein: 4g

29. Eggplant Salad

Preparation Time: 10 minutes

Cooking Time: 30 minutes

Servings: 3

Ingredients: 2 garlic cloves

2 eggplants, peeled and sliced

2 green bell paper, sliced, seeds removed

½ cup fresh parsley

½ cup egg-free mayonnaise

Salt and black pepper

Directions: Preheat your oven to 480 °F Take a baking pan and add the eggplants and black pepper   Bake for about 30 minutes   Flip the vegetables after 20 minutes Then, take a bowl and add baked vegetables and all the remaining ingredients Mix well Serve and enjoy!

Nutrition: Calories: 196

Fat: 108.g Carbohydrates: 13.4g

Protein: 14.6g

30. Cajun Crab

Preparation Time: 10 minutes

Cooking Time: 10 minutes

Servings: 2

Ingredients: 2 bay leaves

1 lemon, fresh and quartered

3 tablespoons Cajun seasoning

4 snow crab legs, precooked and defrosted

Golden ghee

Directions: Take a large pot and fill it about halfway with salted water Bring the water to a boil Squeeze lemon juice into a pot and toss in remaining lemon quarters Add bay leaves and Cajun seasoning Then season for 1 minute Add crab legs and boil for 8 minutes (make sure to keep them submerged the whole time) Melt ghee in the microwave and use as a dipping sauce, enjoy!

Nutrition: Calories: 643

Fat: 51g Carbohydrates: 3g Protein: 41g

31.Mushroom Pork Chops

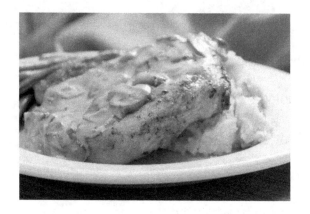

Preparation Time: 10 minutes

Cooking Time: 40 minutes

Servings: 3

Ingredients:

8 ounces mushrooms, sliced

1 teaspoon garlic

1 onion, peeled and chopped

1 cup egg-free mayonnaise

3 pork chops, boneless

1 teaspoon ground nutmeg

1 tablespoon balsamic vinegar

½ cup of coconut oil

Directions:

Take a pan and place it over medium heat

Add oil and let it heat up

Add mushrooms, onions, and stir

Cook for 4 minutes

Add pork chops, season with nutmeg, garlic powder, and brown both sides

Transfer the pan in the oven and bake for 30 minutes at 350 °F

Transfer pork chops to plates and keep it warm

Take a pan and place it over medium heat

Add vinegar, mayonnaise over the mushroom mixture and stir for a few minutes

Drizzle sauce over pork chops

Enjoy!

Nutrition:

Calories: 600

Fat: 10g

Carbohydrates: 8g Protein: 30g

32. Herbed Chicken with Veggies

Preparation Time: 10mins

Cooking Time: 20mins

Servings: 4

Ingredients:

1 - cup sliced carrots, fresh or frozen

2 - cups green beans, fresh or frozen

½ - cup diced onion

8 - bone-in chicken thighs

½ - cup reduced-sodium chicken broth

2 - teaspoons Worcestershire sauce

1 - teaspoon no-salt herb seasoning blend

1 - teaspoon dried oregano

½ - large chicken breast for 1 chicken thigh

Directions:

Spot carrots, green beans, and onions in the moderate cooker.

Mastermind chicken over vegetables.

Pour juices over the chicken, top with Worcestershire sauce, herbs, and flavoring.

Spread and cook on LOW heat for 6 hours.

Present with white rice or rolls.

Nutrition:

Calories: 205 Fat: 6g Protein: 31g Carbs: 5g

33. Roasted Citrus Chicken

Preparation Time: 20mins

Cooking Time: 60mins

Servings: 8

Ingredients 1 - Tablespoon olive oil

2 - cloves garlic, minced

1 - teaspoon Italian seasoning

½ - teaspoon black pepper

8 - chicken thighs

2 - cups chicken broth, reduced-sodium

3 - Tablespoons lemon juice

½ - large chicken breast for 1 chicken thigh

Directions: Warm oil in huge skillet. Include garlic and seasonings.   Include chicken bosoms and dark-colored all sides. Spot chicken in the moderate cooker and include the chicken soup.   Cook on LOW heat for 6 to 8hrs.   Include lemon juice toward the part of the bargain time.

Nutrition: Calories: 265 Fat: 19g Protein: 21g Carbs: 1g

34. Chicken with Asian Vegetables

Preparation Time: 10mins

Cooking Time: 20mins

Servings: 8

Ingredients:

2 - Tablespoons canola oil

6 - boneless chicken breasts

1 - cup low-sodium chicken broth

3 - Tablespoons reduced-sodium soy sauce

¼ - teaspoon crushed red pepper flakes

1 - garlic clove, crushed

1 - can (8ounces) water chestnuts, sliced and rinsed (optional)

½ - cup sliced green onions

1 - cup chopped red or green bell pepper

1 - cup chopped celery

¼ - cup cornstarch

⅓ - cup water

3 - cups cooked white rice

½ - large chicken breast for 1 chicken thigh

Directions:

Warm oil in a skillet and dark-colored chicken on all sides.

Add chicken to slow cooker with the remainder of the fixings aside from cornstarch and water.

Spread and cook on LOW for 6 to 8hrs.

Following 6-8 hours, independently blend cornstarch and cold water until smooth. Gradually include into the moderate cooker.

At that point turn on high for about 15mins until thickened. Don't close top on the moderate cooker to enable steam to leave.

Serve Asian blend over rice.

Nutrition:

Calories: 415 Fat: 20g Protein: 20g Carbs: 36g

35. King Ranch Casserole

Preparation Time: 15mins

Cooking Time: 25mins

Servings: 8

Ingredients:

4 - cups chopped, cooked chicken

1 - large onion, chopped

1 - large green bell pepper, chopped

1 - cup low sodium chicken broth

1 - cup cream of mushroom soup, reduced-sodium

1 - cup canned diced tomatoes, no salt added

1 4 - oz. can green chilies

2 - garlic cloves, minced

2 - teaspoons chili powder

1 - Tablespoon cornstarch plus 1 cup water (stirring until smooth)

12 - (6 inch) corn tortillas

½ - cup shredded sharp cheddar cheese

Directions:

Mix all fixings aside from tortillas and cheddar in an enormous bowl.

Attack 1 inch pieces; separate into thirds. Layer 33% of tortilla pieces in a gently lubed 6 quart moderate cooker.

Top with ⅓ of the chicken blend and about ⅓ of the cheddar.

Rehash layers twice.

Spread and cook on LOW for 3 ½hrs or until bubbly and edges are brilliant dark-colored.

Reveal and cook on LOW for extra 30mins.

Top with acrid cream whenever wanted.

Nutrition:

Calories268 Fat: 7g Protein: 27g Carbs: 25g

36. Southern Chicken and Grits

Preparation Time: 5mins

Cooking Time: 15mins

Servings: 4

Ingredients:

1 ¾ - cups fat-free reduced-sodium chicken broth

6 - Tablespoons corn grits, uncooked

1 - Tablespoon olive oil

1 - small onion, diced

1 - medium clove garlic, minced

1 - cup sliced mushrooms

1 - medium jalapeno pepper, seeded and minced

1 - medium red bell, chopped

¼ - teaspoon ground cumin

¼ - teaspoon black pepper

1 - pound boneless, skinless chicken thighs, cut into 1-inch chunks

Directions:

Spot soup in a 3-to 5-quart moderate cooker. Gradually include cornmeal, mixing continually, to evade irregularities, put the moderate cooker in a safe spot.

Warm oil in an enormous skillet over medium-high heat.

Include onion, garlic, mushrooms, jalapeno, and red pepper; sauté mixing as often as possible, for around 5 minutes.

Add vegetables to slow cooker, alongside cumin and pepper, blend blend.

Include chicken thighs top.

Spread and cook on LOW for 6 to 8hrs.

Nutrition:

Calories259 Fat: 9g Protein: 27g Carbs: 17g

37.   Chicken Adobo

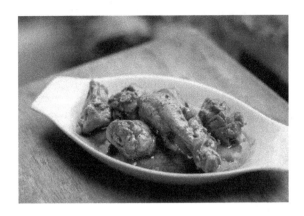

Preparation Time: 10mins

Cooking Time: 1hr 40mins

Servings: 6

Ingredients:

4 - medium yellow onions, halved and thinly sliced

4 - medium garlic cloves, smashed and peeled

1 - (5-inch) piece fresh ginger, cut into

1 - inch pieces

1 - bay leaf

3 - pounds bone-in chicken thighs

3 - Tablespoons reduced-sodium soy sauce

¼ - cup rice vinegar (not seasoned)

1 - Tablespoon granulated sugar

½ - teaspoon freshly ground black pepper

Directions:

Spot the onions, garlic, ginger, and narrows leaf in an even layer in the slight cooker.

Take out and do away with the pores and skin from the chicken.

Organize the hen in an even layer over the onion mixture.

Whisk the soy sauce, vinegar, sugar, and pepper collectively in a medium bowl and pour it over the fowl.

Spread and prepare dinner on LOW for 8hrs.

Evacuate and take away the ginger portions and inlet leaf.

Present with steamed rice.

Nutrition:

Calories318 Fat: 9g Protein: 14g Carbs: 44g

38. Chicken and Veggie Soup

Preparation Time: 15mins

Cooking Time: 25mins

Servings: 8

Ingredients:

4 - cups cooked and chopped chicken

7 - cups reduced-sodium chicken broth

1 - pound frozen white corn

1 - medium onion diced

4 - cloves garlic minced

2 - carrots peeled and diced

2 - celery stalks chopped

2 - teaspoons oregano

2 - teaspoon curry powder

½ - teaspoon black pepper

Directions: Include all fixings into the moderate cooker.Cook on LOW for 8hrs. Serve over cooked white rice.

Nutrition: Calories220 Fat:7g Protein: 24g Carbs: 19g

39. Pesto Chicken

Preparation Time: 5mins

Cooking Time: 30mins

Servings: 6

Ingredients:

3 - chicken breast fillets

6 - ounce jar of pesto

½ - cup of reduced-sodium chicken

Directions:

Spot chicken bosoms at the base of the moderate cooker.

Pour pesto over the chicken and spread to coat the highest points of the chicken.

Pour in ½ cup chicken stock.

Cook on LOW for 6 to 8hrs.

Serve over cooked pasta.

Nutrition:

Calories: 278 Fat: 18g Protein: 28g Carbs: 1g

40. Spicy Coconut Curry Chicken

Preparation Time: 20mins

Cooking Time: 50mins

Servings: 4

Ingredients:

2 - boneless chicken breasts (fresh or frozen)

¼ - cup chopped green onions

1 - (4 ounce) diced green chili peppers

2 - Tablespoons minced garlic

1 ½ - Tablespoons curry powder

1 - Tablespoon chili powder

1 - teaspoon cumin

½ - teaspoon cinnamon

1 - Tablespoon lime juice

1 ½ - cup water

1 - (7 ounce) can coconut milk

1 - cup dry white rice

Chopped cilantro, for garnish

Directions:

Consolidate all fixings except for coconut milk and rice in the moderate cooker.

Spread and cook on LOW for 7-9hrs.

In the wake of cooking time, shred chicken with a fork, mix in coconut milk and dry rice.

Turn the moderate cooker to HIGH and cook for an extra 30mins, or until the rice has consumed the fluid and is cooked.

Serve hot and decorate with cilantro.

Nutrition:

Calories: 270 Fat: 19g Protein: 20g Carbs: 7g

41.Chicken Enchilada Casserole

Preparation Time: 30mins

Cooking Time: 45mins

Servings: 8

Ingredients:

9 - corn tortillas, 6-inch

2 - cups cooked diced chicken

1 to 16 - ounce bag frozen corn

1 - teaspoon chili powder

¼ - teaspoon ground black pepper

1 - can (4 ounces) chopped green chili peppers, mild

1 - cup shredded Mexican blend cheese

1 - cup green chili salsa

1 - can (15 ounces) no sodium black beans, rinsed and drained,

½ - cup sour cream

Directions:

Splash moderate cooker with cooking shower. Spot 3 tortillas in the base of the moderate cooker.

Top tortillas with half of the chicken, the corn, about portion of the seasonings, and half of the stew peppers.

Sprinkle with half of the destroyed cheddar and pour about ½ cup salsa over the cheddar.

Rehash with 3 additional tortillas, the dark beans, staying chicken, seasonings, stew peppers, and cheddar.

Top with outstanding tortillas and salsa.

Spread and cook on LOW for 5 to 6hrs.

Serve warm and can include one Tablespoon of acrid cream on each plate.

Nutrition:

Calories: 308 Fat: 10g Protein: 20g Carbs: 37g

42.   Orange Chicken

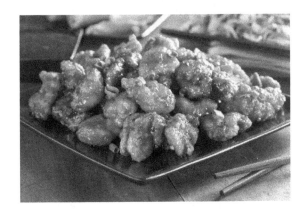

Preparation Time: 10mins

Cooking Time: 13mins

Servings: 8

Ingredients:

8 - bone-in chicken thighs

⅓ - cup flour

1 - tablespoon balsamic vinegar

1 - tablespoon ketchup

4 - ounces orange juice

1 - tablespoon brown sugar

1 - medium onion, chopped

 Medium bell pepper, chopped

Directions:

Spot chicken and flour into a plastic sack, shake to coat.

Add covered chicken to the moderate cooker.

Blend the squeezed orange, dark colored sugar, vinegar, and ketchup into a bowl.

Pour sauce into the moderate cooker over the chicken and blend.

Cook on LOW 6 to 8hrs. Draw chicken off of the bone and serve over white rice with a portion of the sauce.

Nutrition:

Calories: 236 Fat: 15g Protein: 17g Carbs: 8.4g

43. Balsamic Chicken Thighs

Preparation Time: 15mins

Cooking Time: 20mins

Servings: 8

Ingredients: 8 - chicken thighs   - 1 - teaspoon garlic powder

1 - teaspoon dried basil - ½ - teaspoon salt - ½ - teaspoon pepper

2 - teaspoons dried minced onion

4 - garlic cloves, minced - 1 - Tablespoon olive oil - ½ - cup balsamic vinegar

Fresh chopped parsley

Directions: Join the initial 5 dry flavors in a touch bowl and unfold over chicken on the 2 aspects. Put in a secure spot. Pour olive oil and garlic on the base of the moderate cooker. Spot hen on top. Pour balsamic vinegar over the bird. Spread and cook dinner on LOW for 6 to 8hrs. Sprinkle with crisp parsley on top. Serve over noodles.

Nutrition: Calories: 230 Fat: 16g Protein: 16g Carbs: 3g

44. Honey Sesame Chicken

Preparation Time: 10mins

Cook Time: 15mins

Servings: 6

Ingredients: 6 - skinless chicken thighs

1 - Tablespoon olive oil ½ - cup honey

2 - Tablespoon sesame seeds

¼ - cup light low sodium soy sauce

¼ - cup water

1 - Tablespoon sesame oil

1 - teaspoon pepper

1 (10 ounces) package frozen broccoli

Directions: Spot all fixings in a cooler sack, toss to coat.   Spot in the moderate cooker and cook on LOW for 4 to 5hrs.

Take chicken and shred, and after that arrival to the sauce.

Serve over hot cooked rice.

Nutrition: Calories: 247 Fat: 9g Protein: 16g Carbs: 28g

45. Hawaiian Chicken and Rice

Preparation Time: 15mins

Cooking Time: 20mins

Servings: 11

Ingredients:

6 - inch piece ginger, chopped into 1 - inch pieces

2 - medium carrots, chopped into ½ - inch pieces

2 - cup uncooked white rice, rinsed

1 - pound boneless skinless chicken thighs

7 - cups no/low sodium chicken broth

1 - Tablespoon oyster flavored sauce

1 - Tablespoon low sodium soy sauce

1 - Tablespoon sesame oil

1 - small green cabbage, chopped into bite-sized pieces

12 - medium green onions, chopped into 1 - inch pieces

Cilantro

Directions:

Refrigerate hacked cabbage, green onions, and Chinese parsley (discretionary) until prepared to utilize.

In moderate cooker, consolidate ginger, carrots, rice, chicken, and spread with chicken soup.

Spread moderate cooker and cook on LOW for 7 to 9hrs.

During the last 1hr of cooking, open the moderate cooker and blend in cabbage and green onions. Spread and cook for 60 minutes.

Include shellfish sauce, soy sauce, cilantro, and sesame oil into the pot before serving.

Present with canned pineapple whenever wanted

Nutrition:

Calories: 371 Fat: 6g Protein: 25g Carbs: 54g

46. Shredded Chicken Taco Filling

Preparation Time: 15mins

Cooking Time: 15mins

Servings: 10

Ingredients:

2 - cups diced onions

2 ¼ - pounds boneless, skinless chicken breast

½ - cup lime juice

1 - teaspoon ground coriander

2 ½ - teaspoons cumin

2 - teaspoons garlic powder

1 - Tablespoon smoked paprika

1 ½ - teaspoon chili powder

Directions:

With cooking oil try spray the side and bottom of a cooker.

Spot onions on the base of the slight cooker; include chicken, lime squeeze and flavors.

Cook on LOW for 8hrs or until the hen is completed;

Shred chook with 2 forks.

It can serve on flour tortillas and top with lettuce and sharp cream (optional).

Nutrition:

Calories: 117 Fat: 3g Protein: 22g Carbs: 5g

47. Mexican beef flour wrap

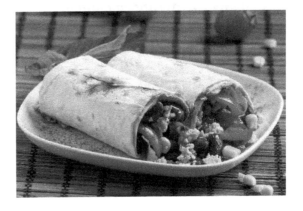

Preparation Time: 10 minutes

Cooking Time: 10 minutes

Servings: 2

Ingredients:

5 oz. Cooked roast beef

8 cucumber slices

2 flour tortillas, 6-inch size

2 tbsp. Whipped cream cheese

2 leaves light green lettuce

1/4 bowl cut red onion

1/4 stripped cut sweet bell pepper

1 tsp. Herb seasoning blend

Directions:

Spread the cheese over the flour wraps. Try to use the ingredients to make two wraps.

Layer the tortillas with roast beef, onions, lettuce, pepper strips and cucumber.

Sprinkle with the herb seasoning

Roll up the wraps and cut them into 4 pieces each. Serve fresh. Enjoy!

Nutrition:

Calories: 255

Protein: 24 g

Sodium: 275 mg

Potassium: 445 mg

Phosphorus: 250 mg

48. Mixed chorizo in egg flour wraps

Preparation Time: 10 minutes

Cooking Time: 10 minutes

Servings: 2

Ingredients:

1 pack chorizo

1 egg

1 flour tortilla or 6-inch size

Direction

Cook the chorizo in a pan on stove, cutting the meat into small pieces.

Eliminate excessive water or fat and add 1 egg combining all while they are being cooked.

Serve everything on a flour tortilla or wrapping the tortillas. Enjoy!

Nutrition: Calories: 223

Protein: 15 g Sodium: 315 mg

Potassium: 285 mg Phosphorus: 230 mg

49. Sandwich with chicken salad

Preparation Time: 10 minutes

Cooking Time: 10 minutes

Servings: 2

Ingredients:

2 bowls cooked chicken

1/2 cup low-fat mayonnaise

1/2 cup green bell pepper

1 cup pieces pineapple

1/3 cup carrots

4 slices flatbread

1/2 tsp. Black pepper

Directions:

Prepare aside the diced chicken and drain pineapple, adding green bell pepper, black pepper and carrots.

Combine all in a bowl and refrigerate until chilled.

Later on, serve the chicken salad on the flatbread. Enjoy!

Nutrition:

Calories: 345

Protein: 22 g

Sodium: 395 mg

Potassium: 330 mg

Phosphorus: 165 mg

Chapter 6: Dinner Recipes

50. Vegetable Confetti Relish

Preparation time: 25 minutes

Cooking time: 15 minutes

Serving: 1

Ingredients:

½ - red bell pepper

½ - green pepper, boiled and chopped

4 - scallions, thinly sliced

½ - tsp. ground cumin

3 - tbsp. vegetable oil

1 ½ - tbsp. white wine vinegar

black pepper to taste

Directions:

Join all fixings and blend well. Chill in the fridge. You can include a large portion of slashed jalapeno pepper for an increasingly fiery blend

Nutrition:

Calories 230,

fat 25,

fiber 3,

carbs 24,

protein 43

51.Chicken and Mandarin Salad

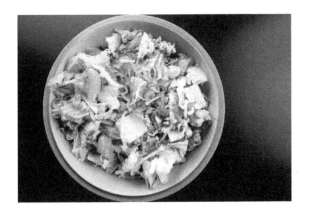

Nutrition:

Calories 375,

fat 15,

fiber 2,

carbs 14,

protein 28

Preparation time: 40 minutes

Cooking time: 30 minutes

Servings: 3

Ingredients:

1 ½ - cup Chicken

½ - cup Celery

½ - cup Green pepper

¼ - cup Onion, finely sliced

1 - cup Mandarin orange segments

¼ - cup Light mayonnaise

½ - tsp. freshly ground pepper

Directions:

Hurl chicken, celery, green pepper and onion to blend. Include mandarin oranges, mayo and pepper. Blend delicately and serve.

52. Roasted Red Pepper Soup

Preparation time: 30 minutes

Cooking time: 35 minutes

Servings: 4

Ingredients:

4 - cups low-sodium chicken broth

3 - red peppers

2 - medium onions

3 - tbsp. lemon juice

1 - tbsp. finely minced lemon zest

A pinch cayenne pepper

¼ - tsp. cinnamon

½ - cup finely minced fresh cilantro

Directions:

In a medium stockpot, consolidate each one of the fixings except for the cilantro and warmth to the point of boiling over excessive warm temperature. Diminish the warmth and stew, ordinarily secured, for around 30 minutes, till thickened. Cool marginally. Utilizing a hand blender or nourishment processor, puree the soup. Include the cilantro and tenderly heat.

Nutrition:

Calories 266,

fat 8,

fiber 6,

carbs 6,

protein 31

53. Leek, Potato and Carrot Soup

Preparation time: 15 minutes

Cooking time: 25 minutes

Servings: 4

Ingredients:

1 - leek

¾ - cup diced and boiled potatoes

¾ - cup diced and boiled carrots

1 - garlic clove

1 - tbsp. oil

crushed pepper to taste

3 - cups low sodium chicken stock

chopped parsley for garnish

1 - bay leaf

¼ - tsp. ground cumin

Directions:

Trim off and take away a portion of the coarse inexperienced portions of the leek, at that factor reduce daintily and flush altogether in virus water. Channel properly. Warmth the oil in an extensively based pot. Include the leek and garlic, and sear over low warmth for two-3 minutes, till sensitive. Include the inventory, inlet leaf, cumin, and pepper. Heat the mixture to the point of boiling, mixing constantly. Include the bubbled potatoes and carrots and stew for 13 minutes. Modify the flavoring, eliminate the inlet leaf and serve sprinkled with slashed parsley. To make a pureed soup, manner the soup in a blender or nourishment processor till smooth. Come again to the pan. Include ½ field milk. Bring to bubble and stew for 4 mins.

Nutrition:

Calories 325,

fat 9,

fiber 5,

carbs 16,

protein 29

54.   Creamy Vinaigrette

Preparation time: 15 minutes

Cooking time: 25 minutes

Servings: 4

Ingredients:

2 - tbsp. cider vinegar

2 - tbsp. lime or lemon juice

1 - garlic clove, minced

1 - tsp. Dijon mustard

1 - tsp. ground cumin

½ - cup sour cream

2 - tbsp. olive oil

¼ - tsp. black pepper

Directions:

Consolidate all fixings and blend well. Fill serving of mixed greens carafe. Chill.

Nutrition: Calories 188,

fat 15,   fiber 8,   carbs 35,

protein 25

55.   Chicken and Pasta Salad

Preparation time: 30 minutes

Cooking time: 25 minutes

Servings: 6

Ingredients:

Chicken Pasta Salad

6 oz. cooked chicken

3 - cups pasta, spiral, cooked

½ - green pepper, minced

1 ½ - tbsp. onion

½ - cup celery

Combine all the above ingredients

Garlic Mustard Vinaigrette

2 - tbsp. cider Vinegar

2 - tsp mustard, prepared

½ - tsp. white sugar

1 - garlic clove, Minced

1/3 - cup water

1/3 - cup olive oil

2 - tsp. parmesan cheese, grated

½ - tsp. ground pepper

Directions:

In a little bowl, combine vinegar, mustard, sugar, garlic, and water; slowly race in oil. Mix in Parmesan. Season with pepper. Join 1/3 measure of dressing with Chicken Pasta Salad and chill.

Nutrition:

Calories 233,

fat 12,

fiber 6,

carbs 25,

protein 23

56. Herbed Soup with Black Beans

Preparation time: 10 minutes

Cooking time: 10 minutes

Servings: 4

Ingredients:

2 tbsp tomato paste

1/3 cup Poblano pepper, charred, peeled, seeded and chopped

2 cups vegetable stock

¼ tsp cumin

½ tsp paprika

½ tsp dried oregano

2 tsp fresh garlic, minced

1 cup onion, small diced

1 tbsp extra-virgin olive oil

1 15-oz can black beans, drained and rinsed

Directions:

On medium fire, place a soup pot and heat oil. Add onion and sauté until translucent and soft, around 4-5 minutes. Add garlic, cook for 2 minutes. Add the rest of the ingredients and bring to a simmer. Once simmering, turn off the fire and transfer to a blender. Puree ingredients until smooth.

Nutrition:

calories 98,

fat 21,

fiber 10,

carbs 20,

protein 19

57. Creamy Pumpkin Soup

Preparation time: 10 minutes

Cooking time: 20 minutes

Servings: 4

Ingredients:

1 onion, chopped

1 slice of bacon

2 tsp ground ginger

1 tsp cinnamon

1 cup applesauce

3 ½ cups low sodium chicken broth

1 29-oz can pumpkin

Pepper to taste

½ cup light sour cream

Directions:

On medium high fire, place a soup pot and add bacon once hot. Sauté until crispy, around 4 minutes. Discard bacon fat, before continuing to cook. Add ginger, applesauce, chicken broth and pumpkin. Lightly season with pepper. Bring to a simmer and cook for 11 minutes. Taste and adjust seasoning. Turn off fire, stir in sour cream and mix well.

Nutrition: calories 220,

fat 8, fiber 10, carbs 36,

protein 10

58. Herbs and Lemony Roasted Chicken

Preparation time: 6 minutes

Cooking time: 11 minutes

Servings: 8

Ingredients:

½ tsp ground black pepper

½ tsp mustard powder

½ tsp salt

1 3-lb whole chicken

1 tsp garlic powder

2 lemons

2 tbsp olive oil

2 tsp Italian seasoning

Directions:

In a small bowl, mix well black pepper, garlic powder, mustard powder, and salt. Rinse chicken well and slice off giblets. In a greased 9 x 13 baking dish, place chicken and add 1 ½ tsp of seasoning made earlier inside the chicken and rub the remaining seasoning around the chicken. In a small bowl, mix olive oil and juice from 2 lemons.

Drizzle over chicken. Bake chicken in a preheated 3500F oven until juices run clear, around 1 ½ hour. Every once in a while, baste the chicken with its juices.

Nutrition: calories 188, fat 9, fiber 6, carbs 20, protein 45

59. Tomato stuffed Portobello Caps

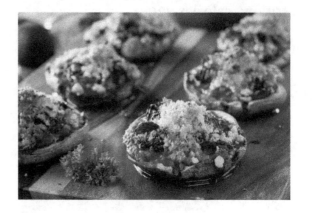

Preparation time: 6 minutes

Cooking time: 11 minutes

Servings: 2

Ingredients:

½ cup mozzarella cheese, shredded

½ tsp rosemary, finely chopped

1 tsp minced garlic

1/8 tsp ground pepper

2 tbsp lemon juice

2 tsp extra virgin olive oil

2 tsp low sodium soy sauce

2/3 cup tomatoes, chopped

4 Portobello mushroom caps

Directions:

Take a bowl and mix tomatoes, cheese, 1 teaspoon olive oil, garlic and pepper. Preheat the grill to medium heat. Discard the stem from the mushrooms. In a small bowl, mix 1 teaspoon olive oil, soy sauce and lemon juice. Brush the insides of the mushroom caps with the oil mixture. Grill the mushroom caps stem sides down and let it cook for five minutes on each side. Remove from the grill and fill with the tomato filling. Top with mozzarella cheese. Return the mushroom to the grill and cook until the cheese has melted.

Nutrition: calories 278, fat 8, fiber 6, carbs 18, protein 20

60. Beef Curry Delight

Preparation time: 10 minutes

Cooking time: 120 minutes

Servings: 6

Ingredients:

2 pounds boneless beef chuck (cut into 1 ½ inch pieces) - 1 cup of water

1 tsp cayenne pepper

1 tsp garlic powder

1 tsp ground turmeric

1 tsp ground coriander

1 tsp ground cumin

1 ½ (2 inches) cinnamon sticks

2 whole cloves

3 whole cardamom seeds

1 tsp ginger paste

5 green Chile peppers (finely sliced)

6 cloves garlic, minced

1 onion, chopped

3 tbsp olive oil

Directions:

Take a skillet, heat the olive oil with medium heat and add the onion. Cook onion for about 6 minutes, once it has softened, reduce heat to medium-low. Then for about 15 to 20 minutes, continue cooking until onion is very tender and dark brown. Stir and cook the cinnamon sticks, cloves, cardamom seeds, ginger paste, green chiles, and garlic. Cook for 3 to 5 minutes until garlic begins to brown. In the onion mixture, add or mix water, cayenne pepper, garlic powder, turmeric, coriander, and cumin. Simmer until the mixture has thickened and until most water has evaporated. For 1 and 1 ½ hours, cook the beef chuck pieces then simmer it over medium-low heat and stir until beef is cooked and tender.

Nutrition: calories 290, fat 10, fiber 11, carbs 8, protein 35

61. Swordfish and Citrus Salsa Delight

Preparation time: 10 minutes

Cooking time: 30 minutes

Servings: 6

Ingredients:

1 ½ pounds swordfish steaks

1 tbsp pineapple juice concentrate (thawed)

¼ tsp cayenne pepper

1 tbsp olive oil

½ cup fresh orange juice

1 tbsp chopped fresh cilantro

2 tsp white sugar

1 tbsp diced red bell pepper

3 tbsp orange juice

2 jalapeno peppers (seeded and minced)

¼ cup diced fresh mango

½ cup canned pineapple chunks (undrained)

1 orange (peeled, and cut into bite-size)

Directions:

In a bowl, make the salsa by combining and mixing well the cilantro, oranges, sugar, pineapple chunks, diced red bell pepper, minced jalapenos, mango, and 3 tablespoons orange juice. Cover the bowl and refrigerate. Mix the pineapple juice concentrate, cayenne pepper, olive oil and ½ cup orange juice in a non-reactive bowl. Add swordfish steaks in the bowl of pineapple juice mixture. Coat and turn well. Ensure to marinate for about 30 minutes. On a gas grill, set heat to medium-high. For 12 to 15 minutes in total, grill the swordfish on both sides then serve with salsa.

Nutrition:

calories 220,

fat 25,

fiber 16,

carbs 15,

protein 35

62. Roasted Halibut with Banana-Orange Relish

Preparation time: 10 minutes

Cooking time: 12 minutes

Servings: 2

Ingredients:

¼ cup cilantro

½ tsp freshly grated orange zest

½ tsp kosher salt, divided

1 lb halibut or any deep-water fish

1 tsp ground coriander, divided into half

2 oranges (peeled, segmented and chopped)

2 ripe bananas, diced

2 tbsp lime juice

Directions:

In a pan, prepare the fish by rubbing ½ tsp coriander and ¼ tsp kosher salt. Place in a baking sheet with cooking spray and bake for 10 minutes inside a 450-degree Fahrenheit preheated oven. Prepare the relish by stirring the orange zest, bananas, chopped oranges, lime juice, cilantro and the rest of the salt and coriander in a medium bowl. Spoon the relish over the roasted fish.

Nutrition:

calories 178,

fat 7,

fiber 6,

carbs 12,

protein 25

63. Lemony Lentil Salad with Salmon

Preparation time: 10 minutes

Cooking time: 0 minutes

Servings: 3

Ingredients:

¼ tsp salt

½ cup chopped red onion

1 cup diced seedless cucumber

1 medium red bell pepper, diced

1/3 cup extra virgin olive oil

1/3 cup fresh dill, chopped

1/3 cup lemon juice

2 15oz cans of lentils

2 7oz cans of salmon, drained and flaked

2 tsp Dijon mustard

Pepper to taste

Directions:

In a bowl, mix, lemon juice, mustard, dill, salt and pepper. Gradually add the oil, bell pepper, onion, cucumber, salmon flakes and lentils. Toss to coat evenly.

Nutrition:

calories 450,

fat 22,

fiber 10,

carbs 62,

protein 55

64. Salad Greens with Roasted Beets

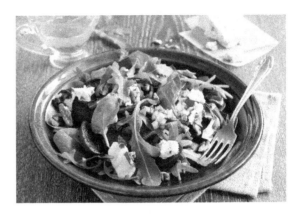

Preparation time: 10 minutes

Cooking time: 60 minutes

Servings: 4

Ingredients:

¼ cup extra-virgin olive oil

½ cup chopped walnuts

½ teaspoon Dijon mustard

1 tablespoon dried cranberries, chopped roughly

1 tablespoon minced red onions

2 tablespoons sherry vinegar

3 medium beets, washed and trimmed

4 cups baby spinach

Directions:

In foil, wrap beets and bake in a preheated 400 F oven. Bake until beets are tender, around 1 hour. Once done, open foil and allow to cool. When cool to touch, peel beets and dice. Mix well mustard, red onions, vinegar, and olive oil. Mix in spinach, beets and cranberries. Toss to coat well.

Nutrition:

calories 180,

fat 15,

fiber 13,

carbs 18,

protein 5

Dinner recipes

65. Eggplant and red pepper soup

Preparation time: 20 minutes

Cooking time: 40 minutes

Servings: 6

Ingredients:

Sweet onion – 1 small, cut into quarters

Small red bell peppers – 2, halved

Cubed eggplant – 2 cups

Garlic – 2 cloves, crushed

Olive oil – 1 tbsp.

Chicken stock – 1 cup

Water

Chopped fresh basil – ¼ cup

Ground black pepper

Directions:

Preheat the oven to 350f.

Put the onions, red peppers, eggplant, and garlic in a baking dish.

Drizzle the vegetables with the olive oil.

Roast the vegetables for 30 minutes or until they are slightly charred and soft.

Cool the vegetables slightly and remove the skin from the peppers.

Puree the vegetables with a hand mixer (with the chicken stock).

Transfer the soup to a medium pot and add enough water to reach the desired thickness.

Heat the soup to a simmer and add the basil.

Season with pepper and serve.

Nutrition:

Calories: 61

Fat: 2g

Carb: 9g

Phosphorus: 33mg

Potassium: 198mg

Sodium: 98mg

Protein: 2g

66.   Seafood casserole

Preparation time: 20 minutes

Cooking time: 45 minutes

Servings: 6

Ingredients:

Eggplant – 2 cups, peeled and diced into 1-inch pieces

Butter, for greasing the baking dish

Olive oil – 1 tbsp.

Sweet onion – ½, chopped

Minced garlic - 1 tsp.

Celery stalk – 1, chopped

Red bell pepper – ½, boiled and chopped

Freshly squeezed lemon juice – 3 tbsp

Hot sauce – 1 tsp.

Creole seasoning mix – ¼ tsp.

White rice – ½ cup, uncooked

Egg – 1 large

Cooked shrimp – 4 ounces

Queen crab meat – 6 ounces

Directions:

Preheat the oven to 350f.

Boil the eggplant in a saucepan for 5 minutes. Drain and set aside.

Grease a 9-by-13-inch baking dish with butter and set aside.

Heat the olive oil in a large skillet over medium heat. Sauté the garlic, onion, celery, and bell pepper for 4 minutes or until tender.

Add the sautéed vegetables to the eggplant, along with the lemon juice, hot sauce, seasoning, rice, and egg

Stir to combine. Fold in the shrimp and crab meat. Spoon the casserole mixture into the casserole dish, patting down the top. 1 Bake for 25 to 30 minutes or until casserole is heated through and rice is tender. 1 Serve warm.

Nutrition: Calories: 118 Fat: 4g

Carb: 9g Phosphorus: 102mg

Potassium: 199mg

Sodium: 235mg Protein: 12g

67. Ground beef and rice soup

Preparation time: 15 minutes

Cooking time: 40 minutes

Servings: 6

Ingredients:

Extra-lean ground beef – ½ pound

Small sweet onion – ½, chopped

Minced garlic – 1 tsp.

Water – 2 cups

Low-sodium beef broth – 1 cup

Long-grain white rice – ½ cup, uncooked

Celery stalk – 1, chopped

Fresh green beans – ½ cup, cut into – 1-inch pieces

Chopped fresh thyme – 1 tsp.

Ground black pepper

Directions:

Sauté the ground beef in a saucepan for 6 minutes or until the beef is completely browned.

Drain off the excess fat and add the onion and garlic to the saucepan.

Sauté the vegetables for about 3 minutes, or until they are softened.

Add the celery, rice, beef broth, and water.

Bring the soup to a boil, reduce the heat to low and simmer for 30 minutes or until the rice is tender.

Add the green beans and thyme and simmer for 3 minutes.

Remove the soup from the heat and season with pepper.

Nutrition: Calories: 154 Fat: 7g

Carb: 14g Phosphorus: 76mg

Potassium: 179mg

Sodium: 133mg Protein: 9g

68.   Couscous burgers

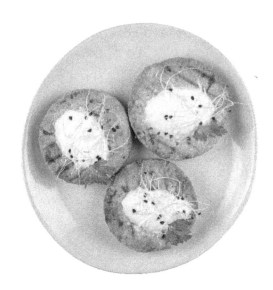

Preparation time: 20 minutes

Cooking time: 10 minutes

Servings: 4

Ingredients:

Canned chickpeas – ½ cup, rinsed and drained

Chopped fresh cilantro – 2 tbsp

Chopped fresh parsley

Lemon juice - 1 tbsp.

Lemon zest – 2 tsp

Minced garlic – 1 tsp.

Cooked couscous – 2 ½ cups

Eggs – 2 lightly beaten

Olive oil – 2 tbsp

Directions:

Put the cilantro, chickpeas, parsley, lemon juice, lemon zest, and garlic in a food processor and pulse until a paste form.

Transfer the chickpea mixture to a bowl and add the eggs and couscous. Mix well. Chill the mixture in the refrigerator for 1 hour. Form the couscous mixture into 4 patties. Heat olive oil in a skillet. Place the patties in the skillet, 2 at a time, gently pressing them down with a spatula. Cook for 5 minutes or until golden and flip the patties over. Cook the other side for 5 minutes and transfer the cooked burgers to a plate covered with a paper towel. Repeat with the remaining 2 burgers.

Nutrition: Calories: 242 Fat: 10g

Carb: 29g Phosphorus: 108mg

Potassium: 168mg

Sodium: 43mg Protein: 9g

69. Baked flounder

Preparation time: 20 minutes

Cooking time: 5 minutes

Servings: 4

Ingredients:

Homemade mayonnaise – ¼ cup

Juice of 1 lime

Zest of 1 lime

Chopped fresh cilantro – ½ cup

Flounder fillets – 4 (3-ounce)

Ground black pepper

Directions:

Preheat the oven to 400f.

In a bowl, stir together the cilantro, lime juice, lime zest, and mayonnaise.

Place 4 pieces of foil, about 8 by 8 inches square, on a clean work surface.

Place a flounder fillet in the center of each square.

Top the fillets evenly with the mayonnaise mixture.

Season the flounder with pepper.

Fold the sides of the foil over the fish, creating a snug packet, and place the foil packets on a baking sheet.

Bake the fish for 4 to 5 minutes.

Unfold the packets and serve.

Nutrition: Calories: 92

Fat: 4g Carb: 2g

Phosphorus: 208mg

Potassium: 137mg

Sodium: 267mg   Protein: 12g

70.   Persian chicken

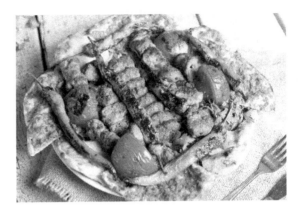

Preparation time: 10 minutes

Cooking time: 20 minutes

Servings: 5

Ingredients:

Sweet onion – ½, chopped

Lemon juice – ¼ cup

Dried oregano – 1 tbsp.

Minced garlic – 1 tsp.

Sweet paprika – 1 tsp.

Ground cumin – ½ tsp.

Olive oil – ½ cup

Boneless, skinless chicken thighs – 5

Directions:

Put the cumin, paprika, garlic, oregano, lemon juice, and onion in a food processor and pulse to mix the ingredients.

Keep the motor running and add the olive oil until the mixture is smooth.

Place the chicken thighs in a large sealable freezer bag and pour the marinade into the bag

Seal the bag and place in the refrigerator, turning the bag twice, for 2 hours.

Remove the thighs from the marinade and discard the extra marinade.

Preheat the barbecue to medium.

Grill the chicken for about 20 minutes, turning once, until it reaches 165f.

Nutrition:

Calories: 321

Fat: 21g

Carb: 3g

Phosphorus: 131mg

Potassium: 220mg

Sodium: 86mg

Protein: 22g

Pork souvlaki

 Preparation time: 20 minutes

cooking time: 12 minutes

servings: 8

Ingredients

Olive oil – 3 tbsp.

Lemon juice – 2 tbsp.

Minced garlic – 1 tsp.

Chopped fresh oregano – 1 tbsp.

Ground black pepper – ¼ tsp.

Pork leg – 1 pound, cut in 2-inch cubes

Directions:

In a bowl, stir together the lemon juice, olive oil, garlic, oregano, and pepper.

Add the pork cubes and toss to coat.

Place the bowl in the refrigerator, covered, for 2 hours to marinate.

Thread the pork chunks onto 8 wooden skewers that have been soaked in water.

Preheat the barbecue to medium-high heat.

Grill the pork skewers for about 12 minutes, turning once, until just cooked through but still juicy.

Nutrition:

Calories: 95

Fat: 4g

Carb: 0g

Phosphorus: 125mg

Potassium: 230mg

Sodium: 29mg

Protein: 13g

71.Pork meatloaf

Preparation time: 10 minutes

Cooking time: 50 minutes

Servings: 8

Ingredients:

95% lean ground beef – 1 pound

Breadcrumbs – ½ cup

Chopped sweet onion – ½ cup

Egg – 1

Chopped fresh basil – 2 tbsp.

Chopped fresh thyme -1 tsp.

Chopped fresh parsley – 1 tsp.

Ground black pepper – ¼ tsp.

Brown sugar – 1 tbsp.

White vinegar – 1 tsp.

Garlic powder – ¼ tsp.

Directions:

Preheat the oven to 350f.

Mix the breadcrumbs, beef, onion, basil, egg, thyme, parsley, and pepper until well combined.

Press the meat mixture into a 9-by-5-inch loaf pan.

In a small bowl, stir together the brown sugar, vinegar, and garlic powder.

Spread the brown sugar mixture evenly over the meat.

Bake the meatloaf for about 50 minutes or until it is cooked through.

Let the meatloaf stand for 10 minutes and then pour out any accumulated grease.

Nutrition:

Calories: 103

Fat: 3g

Carb: 7g

Phosphorus: 112mg

Potassium: 190mg

Sodium: 87mg

Protein: 11g

72.   Chicken stew

Preparation time: 20 minutes

Cooking time: 50 minutes

Servings: 6

Ingredients: Olive oil – 1 tbsp.

Boneless, skinless chicken thighs – 1 pound, cut into 1-inch cubes

Sweet onion – ½, chopped

Minced garlic – 1 tbsp.

Chicken stock – 2 cups

Water – 1 cup, plus 2 tbsp.

Carrot – 1, sliced

Celery – 2 stalks, sliced

Turnip – 1, sliced thin

Chopped fresh thyme – 1 tbsp.

Chopped fresh rosemary – 1 tsp.

Cornstarch – 2 tsp

Ground black pepper to taste

Directions:

Place a large saucepan on medium heat and add the olive oil.

Sauté the chicken for 6 minutes or until it is lightly browned, stirring often.

Add the onion and garlic, and sauté for 3 minutes. Add 1-cup water, chicken stock, carrot, celery, and turnip and bring the stew to a boil. Reduce the heat to low and simmer for 30 minutes or until the chicken is cooked through and tender.

Add the thyme and rosemary and simmer for 3 minutes more.

In a small bowl, stir together the 2 tbsp. Of water and the cornstarch

add the mixture to the stew. Stir to incorporate the cornstarch mixture and cook for 3 to 4 minutes or until the stew thickens. Remove from the heat and season with pepper.

Nutrition: Calories: 141 Fat: 8g

Carb: 5g Phosphorus: 53mg

Potassium: 192mg Sodium: 214mg

Protein: 9g

73.   Beef chili

Preparation time: 10 minutes

Cooking time: 30 minutes

Servings: 2

Ingredients:

Onion – 1, diced

Red bell pepper – 1, diced

Garlic – 2 cloves, minced

Lean ground beef – 6 oz.

Chili powder – 1 tsp.

Oregano – 1 tsp.

Extra virgin olive oil – 2 tbsp.

Water – 1 cup

Brown rice -1 cup

Fresh cilantro – 1 tbsp. To serve

Directions:

Soak vegetables in warm water.

Bring a pan of water to the boil and add rice for 20 minutes.

Meanwhile, add the oil to a pan and heat on medium-high heat.

Add the pepper, onions, and garlic and sauté for 5 minutes until soft.

Remove and set aside.

Add the beef to the pan and stir until browned.

Add the vegetables back into the pan and stir.

Now add the chili powder and herbs and the water, cover and turn the heat down a little to simmer for 15 minutes.

Meanwhile, drain the water from the rice, and the lid and steam while the chili is cooking

Serve hot with the fresh cilantro sprinkled over the top.

Nutrition: Calories: 459

Fat: 22g Carb: 36g Phosphorus: 332mg

Potassium: 360mg Sodium: 33mg

Protein: 22g

74.   Caribbean turkey curry

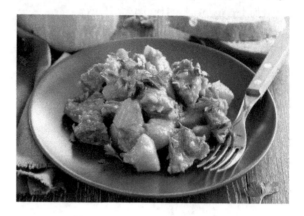

Preparation time: 10 minutes

Cooking time: 1 hour 30 minutes

Servings: 6

Ingredients:

3 1/2 lbs. turkey breast, with skin

1/4 cup butter, melted

1/4 cup honey

1 tbsp mustard

2 tsp curry powder

1 tsp garlic powder

Directions:

Place the turkey breast in a shallow roasting pan.

 Insert a meat thermometer to monitor the temperature. Bake the turkey for 1.5 hours at 350 degrees f until its internal temperature reaches 170 degrees f.

Meanwhile, thoroughly mix honey, butter, curry powder, garlic powder, and mustard in a bowl.

Glaze the cooked turkey with this mixture liberally.

Let it sit for 15 minutes for absorption.

Slice and serve.

Nutrition: calories 275 Protein 26 g

Carbohydrates 9 g Fat 13 g

Cholesterol 82 mg Sodium 122 mg

Potassium 277 mg Phosphorus 193 mg

Calcium 24 mgFiber 0.2 g

75. Lemon and Fruit Pork Kebabs

DIABETES-FRIENDLY, MEDIUM PROTEIN

Preparation time: 20 minutes

Cooking time: 10 minutes

Servings: 4

A plant-based diet prioritizes wholesome plant foods, like fruits and vegetables, at every meal. Most people think of fruit as more of a breakfast or snack food. This dinner recipe incorporates two types of fruit and pairs it with a small amount of pork. These sweet and sour kebabs taste great served alongside a tossed salad or roasted vegetable.

Ingredients:

8 ounces boneless pork loin chops, cubed

1 cup canned pineapple chunks, drained, reserving ¼ cup juice

2 peaches, peeled and cubed

4 scallions, white and green parts, cut into 2-inch pieces

2 tablespoons olive oil

Juice of 1 lemon

2 tablespoons mustard

1 tablespoon cornstarch

2 teaspoons packed brown sugar

Directions

1. Prepare and preheat the grill to medium coals and set a grill 6 inches from the coals.

2. Thread the pork cubes, pineapple, peach cubes, and scallion pieces onto 4 (10-inch) metal skewers. Drizzle the kebabs with olive oil and set aside.

3. In a small saucepan, stir together the reserved pineapple juice, lemon juice, mustard, cornstarch, and brown sugar and bring to a simmer over medium heat. Simmer for 2 to 3 minutes or until the sauce boils and thickens. Remove from heat.

4. Place the kebabs on the grill. Grill for 8 to 10 minutes, turning frequently and brushing with the sauce until the pork registers at least 145°F internal temperature. Use all of the sauce.

5. Remove the kebabs from the heat and let stand for 5 minutes before serving.

Pork can be cooked to medium-well and still be considered food safe. Cook it to at least 145°F, measured with a meat thermometer, and let the pork stand for 5 minutes. This wait time will raise the temperature to 150°F and maintain its juiciness.

Nutrition: Calories: 273; Total fat: 13g; Saturated fat: 3g; Sodium: 118mg; Potassium: 471mg; Phosphorus: 158mg; Carbohydrates: 22g; Fiber: 2g; Protein: 18g; Sugar: 17g

Chapter 7: Dessert Recipe

76.   Cheesecake Bites

Preparation Time: 10 minutes

Cooking Time: 5 minutes

Servings: 16

Ingredients:

8 oz cream cheese

1/2 tsp vanilla

1/4 cup swerve

Directions: Add all ingredients into the mixing bowl and blend until well combined.   Place bowl into the fridge for 1 hour. Remove bowl from the fridge. Make small balls from cheese mixture and place them on a baking dish.   Serve and enjoy.

Nutrition: Calories 50 Fat 4.9 g Carbohydrates 0.4 g Sugar 0.1 g Protein 1.1 g Cholesterol 16 mg

77.   Pumpkin Bites

Preparation Time: 10 minutes

Cooking Time: 5 minutes

Servings: 12

Ingredients: 8 oz cream cheese

1 tsp vanilla   1 tsp pumpkin pie spice

1/4 cup coconut flour   1/4 cup erythritol

1/2 cup pumpkin puree

4 oz butter

Directions: Add all ingredients into the mixing bowl and beat using a hand mixer until well combined. Scoop mixture into the silicone ice cube tray and place it in the refrigerator until set.

Serve and enjoy.

Nutrition: Calories 149 Fat 14.6 g Carbohydrates 8.1 g Sugar 5.4 g Protein 2 g Cholesterol 41 mg

78. Protein Balls

Preparation Time: 5 minutes

Cooking Time: 5 minutes

Servings: 12

Ingredients:

3/4 cup peanut butter

1 tsp cinnamon

3 tbsp erythritol

1 1/2 cup almond flour

Directions:

Add all ingredients into the mixing bowl and blend until well combined.

Place bowl into the fridge for 30 minutes.

Remove bowl from the fridge. Make small balls from mixture and place on a baking dish.

Serve and enjoy.

Nutrition: Calories 179 Fat 14.8 g Carbohydrates 10.1 g Sugar 5.3 g Protein 7 g Cholesterol 0 mg

79. Cashew Cheese Bites

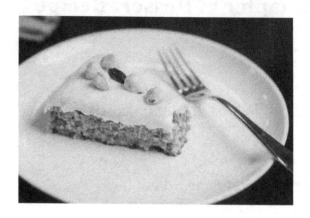

Preparation Time: 5 minutes

Cooking Time: 5 minutes

Servings: 12

Ingredients: 8 oz cream cheese

1 tsp cinnamon

1 cup cashew butter

Directions:

Add all ingredients into the blender and blend until smooth.

Pour blended mixture into the mini muffin liners and place them in the refrigerator until set. Serve and enjoy.

Nutrition: Calories 192 Fat 17.1 g Carbohydrates 6.5 g Sugar 0 g Protein 5.2 g Cholesterol 21 mg

80. Healthy Cinnamon Lemon Tea

Preparation Time: 5 minutes

Cooking Time: 5 minutes

Servings: 1

Ingredients:

1/2 tbsp fresh lemon juice

1 cup of water

1 tsp ground cinnamon

Directions:

Add water in a saucepan and bring to boil over medium heat.

Add cinnamon and stir to cinnamon dissolve.

Add lemon juice and stir well.

Serve hot.

Nutrition: Calories 9 Fat 0.2 g Carbohydrates 2 g Sugar 0.3 g Protein 0.2 g Cholesterol 0 mg

81.Apple Pie

Preparation time: 10 minutes

Cooking time: 50 minutes

Servings: 6

Ingredients:

6 medium apples, peeled, cored & sliced

1/2 cup granulated sugar

1 tsp ground cinnamon

6 tbsp butter

2-2/3 cups all-purpose flour

1 cup shortening

6 tbsp water

Directions

Preheat your oven to 425 degrees F.

Toss the apple slices with cinnamon and sugar in a bowl and set it aside covered.

Blend the flour with the shortening in a pastry blender then add chilled water by the tablespoon.

Continue mixing and adding the water until it forms a smooth dough ball.

Divide the dough into two equal-size pieces and spread them into 2 separate 9-inch sheets.

Arrange the sheet of dough at the bottom of a 9-inch pie pan.

Spread the apples in the pie shell and spread a tablespoon of butter over it.

Cover the filling with the remaining sheet of the dough and pinch down the edges.

Carve 1-inch cuts on top of the pie and bake for 50 minutes or more until golden.

Slice and serve.

Nutrition: Calories 517. Protein 4 g. Carbohydrates 51 g. Fat 33 g. Cholesterol 24 mg. Sodium 65 mg. Potassium 145 mg. Phosphorus 43 mg. Calcium 24 mg. Fiber 2.7 g.

82.   Banana Pudding Dessert

Preparation time: 10 minutes

Cooking time: 5 minutes

Servings: 4

Ingredients: 12 oz vanilla wafers

2 boxes banana cream pudding mix

2-1/2 cups unenriched rice milk

8 oz dairy whipped topping

Directions: Line the bottom of a 9x13 inch pan with a layer of wafers. Mix the banana pudding mix with 2.5 cups of milk in a saucepan.   Bring it to a boil while constantly stirring. Pour this banana pudding over the wafers. Add another layer of wafers over the pudding layer and press them down gently.   Place the layered pudding in the refrigerator for 1 hour. Garnish with whipped cream and serve.

Nutritional Values: Calories 259. Protein 3 g. Carbohydrates 46 g. Fat 7 g. Cholesterol 3 mg. Sodium 276 mg.

Potassium 52 mg. Phosphorus 40 mg. Calcium 9 mg. Fiber 0.3 g.

83. Blueberry Cream Cones

Preparation time: 10 minutes

Cooking time: 0 minutes

Total time: 10 minutes

Servings: 6

Ingredients: 4 oz cream cheese

1-1/2 cup whipped topping

1-1/4 cup fresh or frozen blueberries

1/4 cup blueberry jam or preserves

6 small ice cream cones

Directions

Start by softening the cream cheese then beat it in a mixer until fluffy.

Fold in jam and fruits.

Divide the mixture into the ice cream cones. Serve fresh.

Nutrition: Calories 177. Protein 3 g. Carbohydrates 21 g. Fat 9 g. Cholesterol 21 mg. Sodium 95 mg. Potassium 81 mg. Phosphorus 40 mg. Calcium 24 mg. Fiber 1.0 g.

84. Cherry Coffee Cake

Preparation time: 10 minutes

Cooking time: 40 minutes

Servings: 6

Ingredients:

1/2 cup unsalted butter

2 eggs

1 cup granulated sugar

1 cup sour cream

1 tsp vanilla

2 cups all-purpose white flour

1 tsp baking powder

1 tsp baking soda

20 oz cherry pie filling

Directions:

Preheat oven to 350 degrees F.

Soften the butter first then beat it with the eggs, sugar, vanilla and sour cream in a mixer.

Separately mix flour with baking soda and baking powder.

Add this mixture to the egg mixture and mix well until smooth.

Spread this batter evenly in a 9x13 inch baking pan.

Bake the pie for 40 minutes in the oven until golden on the surface.

Slice and serve with cherry pie filling on top.

Nutrition: Calories 204. Protein 3 g. Carbohydrates 30 g. Fat 8 g. Cholesterol 43 mg. Sodium 113 mg. Potassium 72 mg. Phosphorus 70 mg. Calcium 41 mg. Fiber 0.5 g.

85. Cherry Dessert

Preparation time: 10 minutes

Cooking time: 20 minutes

Total time: 30 minutes

Servings: 6

Ingredients:

1 small package sugar-free cherry gelatin

1 pie crust, 9-inch size

8 oz light cream cheese

12 oz whipped topping

20 oz cherry pie filling

Directions:

Prepare the cherry gelatin as per the given instructions on the packet.

Pour the mixture in an 8x8 inch pan and refrigerate until set.

Soften the cream cheese at room temperature.

Place the 9-inch pie crust in a pie pan and bake it until golden brown.

Vigorously, beat the cream cheese in a mixer until fluffy and fold in whipped topping.

Dice the gelatin into cubes and add them to the cream cheese mixture.

Mix gently then add this mixture to the baking pie shell.

Top the cream cheese filling with cherry pie filling.

Refrigerate for 3 hours then slice to serve.

Nutrition: Calories 258. Protein 5 g. Carbohydrates 28 g. Fat 13 g. Cholesterol 11 mg. Sodium 214 mg. Potassium 150 mg. Phosphorus 50 mg. Calcium 30 mg. Fiber 1.0 g.

86. Crunchy Peppermint Cookies

Preparation time: 10 minutes

Cooking time: 12 minutes

Servings: 6

Ingredients:

1/2 cup unsalted butter

18 peppermint candies

3/4 cup sugar

1 large egg

1/4 tsp peppermint extract

1-1/2 cups all-purpose flour

1 tsp baking powder

Directions:

Soften the butter at room temperature.

Add 12 peppermint candies to a ziplock bag and crush them using a mallet.

Beat butter with egg, sugar and peppermint extract in a mixer until fluffy.

Stir in baking powder and flour and mix well until smooth.

Stir in crushed peppermint candies and refrigerate the dough for 1 hour.

Meanwhile, layer a baking sheet with parchment paper.

Preheat the oven to 350 degrees F.

Crush the remaining candies and keep them aside.

Make ¾-inch balls out of the dough and place them on the baking sheet.

Sprinkle the crushed candies over the balls.

Bake them for 12 minutes until slightly browned.

Serve fresh and enjoy.

Nutrition: Calories 150. Protein 2 g. Carbohydrates 22 g. Fat 6 g. Cholesterol 24 mg. Sodium 67 mg. Potassium 17 mg. Phosphorus 24 mg. Calcium 20 mg. Fiber 0.2 g.

87.   Cranberries Snow

Preparation time: 10 minutes

Cooking time: 12 minutes

Total time: 22 minutes

Servings: 4

Ingredients:

1 cup cran-cherry juice

12 oz fresh cranberries

2 packets gelatin

2 cups granulated sugar

1 cup crushed pineapple, canned in juice

8 oz cream cheese

3 cups whipped topping

Directions:

Boil the cran-cherry juice in a saucepan.

Stir in cranberries and cook for 12 minutes.

Remove the pan from the stove heat and add 1 ¼ cup sugar and gelatin.

Mix well until dissolved then allow it to cool for 30 minutes.

Toss in drained pineapple and mix well then pour it all into a 9x13 inch pan.

Refrigerate this mixture for 1 hour.

Prepare the snow topping by mixing the ¾ sugar and cream cheese in a mixer.

Spread this mixture over the refrigerated cranberry mixture.

Serve fresh.

Nutrition: Calories 210. Protein 2 g. Carbohydrates 35 g. Fat 7 g. Cholesterol 23 mg. Sodium 58 mg. Potassium 65 mg. Phosphorus 25 mg. Calcium 28 mg. Fiber 1.0 g.

88. Chia Pudding with Berries

Preparation time: 10 minutes

Cooking time: 0 minutes

Servings: 4

Ingredients: 1/2 cup chia seeds

2 cups vanilla almond milk, sweetened

1/4 cup shredded sweetened coconut

1/4 cup fresh blueberries

4 large strawberries

Directions:

Blend the almond milk with chia seeds in a blender. Divide this mixture into the serving bowls. Refrigerate them for 1 hour then top them with a strawberry, blueberries and coconut shreds. Serve fresh.

Nutrition: Calories 184. Protein 4 g. Carbohydrates 22 g. Fat 9 g. Cholesterol 0 mg. Sodium 94 mg. Potassium 199 mg. Phosphorus 200 mg. Calcium 362 mg. Fiber 8 g.

89. Vanilla Delight

Preparation time: 10 minutes

Cooking time: 25 minutes

Servings: 15

Ingredients:

1 cup all-purpose white flour

1 stick unsalted margarine

8 oz light cream cheese

8 oz whipped topping

1 cup granulated sugar

4 cartons vanilla pudding

1 tsp vanilla extract

1/2 cup shredded coconut, sweetened

Directions:

Preheat oven to 350 degrees F.

Mix the flour with margarine then spread it in a 9x13 inch pan.

Bake this crust for 25 minutes until golden brown then allows it to cool.

Beat the cream cheese with half of the whipped topping and sugar in a mixer.

Spread this mixture in the baked crust.

Mix pudding with vanilla extract in a separate bowl.

Spread the mixture over the cream cheese filling.

Garnish with the other half of the whipped topping.

Sprinkle coconut on top and refrigerate for 30 minutes.

Slice and serve.

Nutrition: Calories 232. Protein 3 g. Carbohydrates 30 g. Fat 11 g. Cholesterol 7 mg. Sodium 112 mg. Potassium 58 mg. Phosphorus 40 mg. Calcium 101 mg. Fiber 0.4 g.

90.   Strawberry Pie

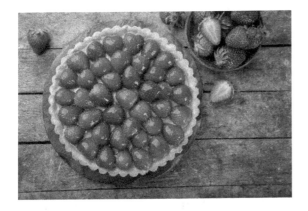

Preparation time: 10 minutes

Cooking time: 25 minutes

Servings: 8

Ingredients:

1 unbaked pie shell, 9" size

4 cups strawberries, fresh or frozen

1 cup of sugar

3 tbsp cornstarch

2 tbsp lemon juice

8 tbsp whipped topping

Directions:

Spread the pie shell in the pie pan and bake it until golden brown.

Now, mash 2 cups strawberries with lemon juice, cornstarch, and sugar in a bowl.

Add this mixture to a saucepan and cook on medium heat until it thickens.

Allow the mixture to cool then spread it in the pie shell.

Slice the remaining strawberries and spread them over the pie filling.

Refrigerate for 1 hour then garnish with whipped cream.

Serve fresh and enjoy.

Nutrition: Calories 212. Protein 1 g. Carbohydrates 40 g. Fat 5.4 g. Cholesterol 15 mg. Sodium 104 mg. Potassium 141 mg. Phosphorus 24 mg. Calcium 20 mg. Fiber 2.0 g.

91. Grapefruit Sorbet

Preparation Time: 10 Minutes

Cooking Time: 5 Minutes

Servings: 6

Many people say that sorbet can't be done without an ice cream maker, but this recipe proves otherwise. Using just four ingredients, you can create this sweet-and-sour showstopper with just a couple of hours' freezing time. Note: This recipe doubles the amount of simple syrup you'll need. You can refrigerate the remaining syrup to make more sorbet within two weeks.

Ingredients:

FOR THE THYME SIMPLE SYRUP

½ cup of sugar

¼ cup of water

1 fresh thyme sprig

FOR THE SORBET

Juice of 6 pink grapefruit

¼ cup thyme simple syrup

Directions:

TO MAKE THE THYME SIMPLE SYRUP

In a small saucepan, combine the sugar, water, and thyme. Bring to a boil, turn off the heat, and refrigerate, thyme sprig included, until cold. Strain the thyme sprig from the syrup.

TO MAKE THE SORBET

1In a blender, combine the grapefruit juice and ¼ cup of simple syrup, and process.

2Transfer to an airtight container and freeze for 3 to 4 hours, until firm. Serve.

Try this with other citrus fruits, such as oranges, lemons, or limes, for an equally delicious treat.

Nutrition: 109; Total Fat: 0g; Saturated Fat: 0g; Cholesterol: 0mg; Carbohydrates: 26g; Fiber: 0g; Protein: 1g; Phosphorus: 29mg; Potassium: 318mg; Sodium: 2mg

92. Zesty Shortbread Cookies

Preparation Time: 10 Minutes

Cooking Time: 15 Minutes

Servings: 16

Shortbread cookies are sweet biscuits perfect for eating out of hand or for dipping in tea. They're also surprisingly easy to make from scratch. Using lime and lemon zest enlivens and elevates these simple snappy treats.

Ingredients:

1 cup all-purpose flour

½ cup powdered sugar, plus more for shaping cookies

½ cup unsalted butter, cut into ½-inch cubes

Zest of 1 lime

Zest of 1 lemon

Directions:

1Preheat the oven to 375°F.

2In a food processor, add the flour, sugar, butter, and lime and lemon zest. Process until the dough just comes together.

3Measure a tablespoon of dough, and use your hands to roll it into a ball. Place on a baking sheet, and continue to roll the dough balls until all of the dough is used up.

4Dip the bottom of a measuring cup into powdered sugar, and press the balls flat with the measuring cup.

5Bake for 13 to 15 minutes, until the edges are just browned. Transfer the cookies to a wire rack to cool. Store in an airtight container for up to five days.

You can dust the cookies with a little more powdered sugar after cooking, but while still hot, if desired.

Nutrition: 94; Total Fat: 6g; Saturated Fat: 4g; Cholesterol: 15mg; Carbohydrates: 10g; Fiber: 0g; Protein: 1g; Phosphorus: 10mg; Potassium: 10mg; Sodium: 1mg

93.   Berry Crumble

Preparation Time: 5 Minutes

Cooking Time: 1 Hour

Servings: 12

This crumble customizes with whatever berries you have on hand, making it perfect for cleaning out your freezer and using the last of your seasonal berries. Mix this topping in just minutes, transfer it to the oven, and in a short hour, you'll have a dessert to drool over. Let it cool for about 30 minutes to allow the juices to thicken slightly before serving.

Ingredients:

6 cups frozen berries (strawberries, raspberries, blueberries, or blackberries)

¼ cup of sugar

¾ cup all-purpose flour

¾ cup rolled oats

¼ cup brown sugar

1 teaspoon ground cinnamon

¼ cup unsalted butter, melted

Directions:

1Preheat the oven to 375°F.

2In a large bowl, toss the berries with the sugar. Transfer to a medium baking dish. 3In the same bowl, add the flour, oats, brown sugar, and cinnamon, and stir well. Pour the melted butter over the mixture, and stir to blend. 4Using your hands, press the mixture together into pieces, and place the clumps over the berries in the baking dish. 5Bake for 1 hour, until the top, is crisp and browned and the berries are bubbling. Let stand for 30 minutes before serving. Substitution tip: You can use pretty much any fruit in a crumble with excellent results. Apples, peaches, pears, and plums also work great.

Per Serving Calories: 167; Total Fat: 5g; Saturated Fat: 3g; Cholesterol: 10mg; Carbohydrates: 29g; Fiber: 4g; Protein: 3g; Phosphorus: 75mg; Potassium: 155mg; Sodium: 3mg

94.   Grape Skillet Galette

Preparation Time: 15 Minutes, Plus 2 Hours To Chill

Cooking Time: 25 Minutes

Servings: 6

A galette may sound fancy, but it's simply a rustic pie made in a free-form style. This makes the crust very forgiving, and you don't have to spend a ton of time rolling the dough and working to make it look picture-perfect. With just one bottom crust, folded inward to cover the fillings, the galette looks and tastes great with little effort.

Ingredients:

FOR THE CRUST

1 cup all-purpose flour

1 tablespoon sugar

4 tablespoons cold butter, cut into ½-inch cubes

½ cup homemade rice milk or unsweetened store-bought rice milk

FOR THE GALETTE

⅓ cup of sugar

1 tablespoon cornstarch

2 cups halved seedless grapes

1 egg white

Directions:

TO MAKE THE CRUST

1In a food processor, add the flour and sugar and pulse a few times to mix. Add the butter, and pulse several times until it resembles a coarse meal. Add the rice milk, and mix until the dough starts to come together.

2Transfer the dough to a clean surface, and shape into a flat disc. Wrap in plastic wrap, and refrigerate for 2 hours or overnight.

TO MAKE THE GALETTE

1Preheat the oven to 425°F.

2In a medium bowl, mix the sugar and cornstarch. Add the grapes, tossing to blend.

3Unwrap the dough and place it on a clean, floured surface. Roll it out into a 14-inch circle and transfer to an oven-safe skillet.

4Add the grape filling in the center of the dough, spreading it outward, leaving a border of about 2 inches of crust. Fold the edges of the dough inward to partially cover the grapes.

5Brush the dough with the egg white. Cook for 20 to 25 minutes, until the crust, is golden. Let rest for at least 20 minutes before serving.

If you don't have an oven-safe skillet, use a large rimmed baking sheet instead. To make cleanup easier, line it with a sheet of parchment paper.

Nutrition: 172; Total Fat: 6g; Saturated Fat: 4g; Cholesterol: 15mg; Carbohydrates: 27g; Fiber: 1g; Protein: 2g; Phosphorus: 21mg; Potassium: 69mg; Sodium: 65mg

95.   Lemon Tart

Preparation Time: 10 Minutes, Plus 30 Minutes To Chill

Cooking Time: 30 Minutes

Servings: 10

If you're a fan of the lively lemon flavor in desserts, this sweet treat will hit the spot. Because it is rich in butter and sugar, the serving is small, but it packs a giant punch of both sour and sweet that is so pleasing. The no-roll tart shell streamlines prep time and ensures great results every time.

Ingredients:

FOR THE TART SHELL

2 tablespoons sugar

1¼ cups all-purpose flour

8 tablespoons unsalted butter, melted

FOR THE TART

½ cup freshly squeezed lemon juice

Zest of 1 lemon

3 large eggs

½ cup of sugar

4 tablespoons butter, cut into pieces

1 lemon, sliced, for garnish

Powdered sugar, for garnish

Directions:

TO MAKE THE TART SHELL

1In a small bowl, whisk the sugar and flour together. Drizzle with the melted butter and stir to blend.

2Transfer the flour mixture to a tart pan, and use your hands to press the dough to the bottom and sides of the pan. Cover with plastic wrap and refrigerate for 30 minutes.

3Preheat the oven to 350°F.

4Prick the tart shell with a fork about 20 times all over, then bake for 20 minutes, until golden brown. Remove from the oven, and cool completely before filling.

TO MAKE THE TART

1In a medium saucepan over medium-high heat, bring the lemon juice and zest to a boil. Remove the pan from the heat.

2In a small bowl, whisk the eggs and sugar together. Slowly pour the egg mixture into the lemon juice, whisking constantly. Cook over medium heat, stirring continually until the mixture has thickened, about 6 to 8 minutes.

3Add the butter pieces, and remove the pan from the heat. Stir until all the butter melts. Strain the custard through a wire mesh strainer into the tart shell. Refrigerate for about 2 hours, until cold, before serving. 4Top with the lemon slices and powdered sugar. Serve.

If you like lemon tart, you can also try the same recipe using limes. Key limes have the most flavor, but the standard grocery-store variety creates a great tart as well.

Nutrition: 252; Total Fat: 15g; Saturated Fat: 5g; Cholesterol: 77mg; Carbohydrates: 25g; Fiber: 1g; Protein: 4g; Phosphorus: 55mg; Potassium: 59mg; Sodium: 29mg

96.   Strawberry Pie

Preparation Time: 10 Minutes

Cooking Time: 20 Minutes

Servings: 8

Strawberry pie conjures visions of a summer picnic, and this one's made with a graham cracker–crumb crust, so there is less fat in the final treat than in one made with a traditional piecrust. This is a fresh pie, meaning the strawberries are not cooked, giving the finished product a fresh, straight-from-the-field flavor.

Ingredients:

FOR THE CRUST

5 tablespoons unsalted butter, at room temperature

2 tablespoons sugar

1½ cups graham-cracker crumbs

FOR THE PIE

5 cups sliced strawberries, divided

¾ cup of sugar

3 tablespoons cornstarch

1½ teaspoons gelatin powder

1 cup of water

Directions:

TO MAKE THE CRUST

1Preheat the oven to 375°F. Grease a pie pan.

2In a small bowl, mix the butter, sugar, and graham cracker crumbs. Press the mixture into the pie pan.

3Bake for 10 to 15 minutes, until lightly browned. Remove from the oven and let cool completely.

TO MAKE THE PIE

1In a small bowl, crush 1 cup of strawberries. 2In a small saucepan, combine the sugar, cornstarch, gelatin, and water. Bring to a boil, reduce the heat, and simmer until the sauce thickens. Add the cup of crushed strawberries, and simmer for another 5 minutes, until the sauce thickens again. Remove from the heat, and transfer to a bowl. Cool to room temperature. 3Toss the remaining 4 cups of berries with the sauce to coat, and pour into the pie shell, spreading in an even layer. Refrigerate until cold, about 3 hours, and serve. To save time, you can buy a ready-made graham cracker–crumb crust from the store.

Nutrition: 265; Total Fat: 9g; Saturated Fat: 5g; Cholesterol: 19mg; Carbohydrates: 45g; Fiber: 3g; Protein: 3g; Phosphorus: 44mg; Potassium: 183mg; Sodium: 143mg

97. Chocolate Beet Cake

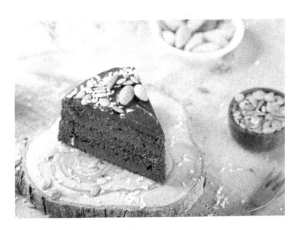

Preparation time: 10 minutes

Cooking time: 50 minutes

Servings: 12

Beets in chocolate cake? Yes! Beets are a nutritional powerhouse, and while adding them to your dessert may seem strange at first, the beet flavor is nearly undetectable, and all you'll taste is the comforting, chocolaty goodness that chocolate cake is known for.

Ingredients: 1 cup of sugar

2 cups all-purpose flour 4 large eggs

2 teaspoons Phosphorus baking powder

4 ounces unsweetened chocolate

¼ cup canola oil 3 cups grated beets

Directions:

1. Preheat the oven to 325°F. Grease two 8-inch cake pans.

2. In a large bowl, whisk the sugar, flour, and baking powder together. Set aside.

3. Finely chop the chocolate, and melt in a double boiler. Let cool, and mix with the eggs and oil. Add the wet ingredients to the dry, mixing well to blend. Fold in the beets, and pour the batter into the cake pans.

4. Bake for 40 to 50 minutes, until a knife inserted in the center of the cake comes out clean. Remove from the oven, and let cool. Invert over a plate to remove.

This cake is great on its own or topped with a bit of whipped cream and fresh berries. Just let the cake cool completely before topping.

Nutrition: 270; Total Fat: 12g; Saturated Fat: 4g; Cholesterol: 70mg; Carbohydrates: 39g; Fiber: 3g; Protein: 6g; Phosphorus: 111mg; Potassium: 299mg; Sodium: 109mg

98. Instant Peach Melba Sorbet

5-INGREDIENT, HIGH FIBER, LOW PROTEIN

Preparation time: 15 minutes

Cooking time: 10 minutes

Servings: 4

This recipe for instant sorbet is somewhat like a smoothie, but much richer in fruit so it is firm and ready to eat as soon as it's blended. You will need a powerful food processor or blender to make this recipe because the frozen fruit can be very hard. If you make this dessert ahead, transfer it to a loaf pan, cover, and freeze up to 3 days. Let the sorbet stand at room temperature for 10 minutes before serving, so it's easier to scoop.

Ingredients:

2 cups frozen peach slices

1 cup frozen raspberries

½ cup plain whole-milk yogurt

1 tablespoon honey

1 teaspoon vanilla

Directions:

1. Combine the peaches, raspberries, yogurt, honey, and vanilla in a food processor or blender. Process or blend until the mixture is smooth; this will take a few minutes. Put a towel over the processor to help muffle the noise.

2. Serve immediately or cover and freeze for a few hours before serving.

To make this a diabetes-friendly recipe, replace the honey with 1 to 2 tablespoons of powdered erythritol. The sugar content will decrease to 10g per serving.

Nutrition: 100; Total fat: 1g; Saturated fat: less than 1g; Sodium: 19mg; Potassium: 270mg; Phosphorus: 60mg; Carbohydrates: 21g; Fiber: 6g; Protein: 2g; Sugar: 15g

99. Thyme and Pineapple Crisp

HIGH FIBER, LOW PROTEIN

Preparation time: 15 minutes

Cooking time: 10 minutes

Servings: 6

A crisp is a dessert made with some kind of fruit base and a crunchy topping with oats and brown sugar. Ordinarily, a crisp would need a minimum of an hour in the oven, but this version cuts that time by sautéing the pineapple in a saucepan and making the topping separately in a skillet.

Ingredients:

1 (20-ounce) can pineapple tidbits in juice, drained, reserving ⅓ cup juice

¼ cup brown sugar, divided

1 tablespoon cornstarch

½ teaspoon dried thyme leaves

3 tablespoons unsalted butter

1¼ cups quick-cooking oats

⅓ cup whole-wheat flour

Pinch salt

2 tablespoons chopped walnuts

Directions:

1. Stir together the drained pineapple, reserved pineapple juice, 1 tablespoon brown sugar, cornstarch, and the thyme leaves in a medium saucepan over medium heat.

2. Cook for 8 to 10 minutes, stirring occasionally until the mixture is thickened.

3. Meanwhile, combine the remaining 3 tablespoons brown sugar and butter in a medium skillet over medium heat, stirring frequently, until the mixture melts.

4. Add the oats, flour, salt, and walnuts to the brown sugar mixture in the skillet.

5. Cook, stirring frequently until the mixture is a deep golden brown, about 5 minutes. Transfer the oat mixture to a plate.

6. When the pineapple mixture is thickened, top with the oatmeal mixture right in the saucepan and serve.

You can use pineapple chunks or even crushed pineapple in this recipe. Just be sure to drain it well before you start.

Choose a pineapple that is canned in juice, not syrup, or the sugar content will be much higher.

Nutrition: Calories: 238; Total fat: 9g; Saturated fat: 4g; Sodium: 31mg; Potassium: 221mg; Phosphorus: 109mg; Carbohydrates: 39g; Fiber: 3g; Protein: 4g; Sugar: 20g

100. Big Peanut Butter Macadamia Cookie

HIGH FIBER, MEDIUM PROTEIN

Preparation time: 15 minutes

Cooking time: 15 minutes

Servings: 4

How fun is it to make one big cookie and let everyone break off a piece? You will feel like you are at a party! This cookie is much faster to make than individual smaller cookies and is delicious served warm. The buttery macadamia nuts are used instead of chopped peanuts to reduce the potassium content of this recipe.

Ingredients:

2 tablespoons unsalted butter

3 tablespoons peanut butter

⅓ cup brown sugar

1 large egg

1 large egg yolk

½ teaspoon vanilla

⅓ cup all-purpose flour

⅓ cup whole-wheat flour

¼ teaspoon Low Phosphorus Baking Powder

2 tablespoons chopped macadamia nuts

Directions:

1.Preheat the oven to 350°F. Line a baking sheet with parchment paper and set aside.

2. In a medium microwave-safe bowl, melt the butter on high power for 30 seconds.

3. Stir in the peanut butter, brown sugar, egg, egg yolk, and vanilla until smooth.

4. Add the all-purpose flour, whole-wheat flour, and baking powder and mix until just combined.

5. Form the dough into a 5-inch round on the parchment paper and sprinkle with the macadamia nuts.

6. Bake for 14 to16 minutes or until the cookie is set and light golden brown. Serve warm.

To reduce the sodium in this recipe to 52 milligrams, you can use unsalted peanut butter. To make this recipe diabetes-friendly, replace the sugar with ⅓ cup plus 1 tablespoon of powdered erythritol. The sugar content will decrease to 2g per serving.

Nutrition: Calories: 323; Total fat: 17g; Saturated fat: 6g; Sodium: 171mg; Potassium: 249mg; Phosphorus: 134mg; Carbohydrates: 36g; Fiber: 2g; Protein: 8g; Sugar: 19g

Chapter 8: 21-Day Kidney Diet Plan

Diets are easier when you have a definitive meal plan in your hands. This 21-day meal plan specifically for the renal diet will help you enjoy all the flavors and nutrients found in this cookbook easily.

Day 01:

Breakfast: Apple Onion Omelet

Lunch: Chicken Wild Rice Soup

Snack: Chicken Pepper Bacon Wraps

Dinner: Braised Beef Brisket

Dessert: Banana Pudding Dessert

Day 02:

Breakfast: Apple Fritter Rings

Lunch: Chicken Noodle Soup

Snack: Snack: Chicken Pepper Bacon Wraps

Dinner: California Pork Chops

Dessert: Blueberry Cream Cones

Day 03:

Breakfast: Apple Cinnamon Maple Granola

Lunch: Cucumber Soup

Snack: Buffalo Chicken Dip

Dinner: Beef Chorizo

Dessert: Cherry Dessert

Day 04:

Breakfast: Asparagus and Cheese Crepe Rolls with Parsley

Lunch: Squash and Turmeric Soup

Snack: Shrimp Spread with Crackers

Dinner: Pork Fajitas

Dessert: Cherry Coffee Cake

Day 05:

Breakfast: Acai Berry Smoothie Bowl

Lunch: Wild Rice Asparagus Soup

Snack: Garlic Oyster Crackers

Dinner: Caribbean Turkey Curry

Dessert: Strawberry Pie

Day 06:

Breakfast: Baked Egg Cups

Lunch: Nutmeg Chicken Soup

Snack: Addictive Pretzels

Dinner: Chicken with Rosemary-Garlic Sauce

Dessert: Vanilla Delight

Day 07:

Breakfast: Belgian Waffles

Lunch: Hungarian Cherry Soup

Snack: Sweet and Spicy Tortilla Chips

Dinner: Chicken Fajitas

Dessert: Chia Pudding with Berries

Day 08:

Breakfast: Clam Omelet

Lunch: Italian Wedding Soup

Snack: Spicy Corn Bread

Dinner: Chicken with Rosemary-Garlic Sauce

Dessert: Cranberries Snow

Day 09:

Breakfast: Confetti Omelet

Lunch: Old Fashioned Salmon Soup

Snack: Sweet Savory Meatballs

Dinner: Chicken Paprika

Dessert: Crunchy Peppermint Cookies

Day 10:

Breakfast: Cottage Cheese Sour Cream Pancakes

Lunch: Oxtail Soup

Snack: Apple Cranberry Slaw

Dinner: Grilled Chicken Marsala

Dessert: Apple Pie

Day 11:

Breakfast: Apple Onion Omelet

Lunch: Pork Fajitas

Snack: Asian Cabbage Slaw

Dinner: Old Fashioned Salmon Soup

Dessert: Cherry Dessert

Day 12:

Breakfast: Apple Fritter Rings

Lunch: Caribbean Turkey Curry

Snack: Autumn Orzo Salad

Dinner: Oxtail Soup

Dessert: Banana Pudding Dessert

Day 13:

Breakfast: Apple Cinnamon Maple Granola

Lunch: Chicken Fajitas

Snack: Basil-Lime Pineapple Salad

Dinner: Italian Wedding Soup

Dessert: Blueberry Cream Cones

Day 14:

Breakfast: Asparagus and Cheese Crepe Rolls with Parsley

Lunch: Chicken with Rosemary-Garlic Sauce

Snack: Basil-Lime Pineapple Salad

Dinner: Hungarian Cherry Soup

Dessert: Cherry Coffee Cake

Day 15:

Breakfast: Acai Berry Smoothie Bowl

Lunch: Chicken Paprika

Snack: Creamy Cucumber Salad

Dinner: Nutmeg Chicken Soup

Dessert: Blueberry Cream Cones

Day 16:

Breakfast: Baked Egg Cups

Lunch: Grilled Chicken Marsala

Snack: Cucumber-Carrot Salad

Dinner: Squash and Turmeric Soup

Dessert: Cherry Coffee Cake

Day 17:

Breakfast: Belgian Waffles

Lunch: Baked Pork Chops

Snack: Garden Vegetable Salad

Dinner: Squash and Turmeric Soup

Dessert: Banana Pudding Dessert

Day 18:

Breakfast: Clam Omelet

Lunch: Braised Beef Brisket

Snack: Green Pepper Slaw

Dinner: Cucumber Soup

Dessert: Apple Pie

Day 19:

Breakfast: Confetti Omelet

Lunch: California Pork Chops

Snack: Cranberry Cream Salad

Dinner: Chicken Noodle Soup

Dessert: Strawberry Pie

Day 20:

Breakfast: Apple Onion Omelet

Lunch: Baked Pork Chops

Snack: Creamy Cucumber Salad

Dinner: Chicken Wild Rice Soup

Dessert: Vanilla Delight

Day 21:

Breakfast: Cottage Cheese Sour Cream Pancakes

Lunch: Squash and Turmeric Soup

Snack: Cucumber-Carrot Salad

Dinner: Baked Pork Chops

Dessert: Apple Pie

Kitchen Staples:

Spices and Herbs:

- Oregano
- Thyme
- Onion powder
- Garlic powder
- Paprika
- Cayenne pepper
- Black pepper
- Chili powder
- Cumin
- Basil
- Rosemary

Vegetables:

- Onion
- Garlic
- Carrots
- Celery
- Bell peppers
- Beets
- Cucumbers
- Peas

Fruits:

- Apples
- Pineapples
- Blueberries

- Strawberries
- Raspberries
- Cranberries
- Banana

Meat and poultry:

- Pork chops
- Beef Briskets
- Chicken legs
- Chicken breasts
- Turkey breasts
- Oysters

Dairy and Non Dairy Items:

- Yogurt
- Cheese
- Low-Fat milk
- Rice milk

Miscellaneous:

- Chia seeds
- Flour
- Sesame seeds (black and white)
- Sesame oil
- Olive oil
- Cherry pie filling
- Pie Crusts
- Green beans
- Butter

- Sweet sauce

- Hot sauce

- Splenda

- Oyster crackers

- Tortilla

- Low sodium bouillon cubes

- Wild rice

- Eggs

Conclusion

Taking care of your kidneys is vital to a healthy life. You have to provide a healthy environment for your kidneys to prevent further cell damage and possible kidney disease. A proper renal diet like the one explained in this cookbook can help you improve or maintain your kidney health to do this by cutting down on the minerals that destabilize the internal balance of your kidneys: sodium, potassium, and phosphorus.

In this cookbook, we tried to offer you the best possible renal diet recipes for everyday consumption ranging from breakfasts to side dishes, snacks, soups, salads, smoothies, meat, and desserts. Equipped with nutritional info and low sodium ingredients, each recipe is worth a try. For additional help, feel free to follow (or modify) the included 21-day meal plan made up of recipes found in the cookbook.

Chapter 9: Getting Used to Low-Sodium Diet Regimen

To get used to lower intake of sodium as well as it should be the case with low intake of potassium, we have compiled a list of tips that should help you find healthier substitutes and alternatives to food groups and condiments that normally contain high levels of sodium. Getting used to a new diet regimen can be difficult at the beginning, but these tips should help you make a successful transition to a healthier diet - renal diet – by slowly and steadily removing high-sodium and high-potassium foods.

Tip #1: Lemon Juice is Your Friend

Did you know that you can use lemon juice as a substitute for salt in your meals? Salt has extremely high concentrations of salt where a single teaspoon of salt may contain your entire daily dose of salt. By using lemon juice for your meals, you will be able to season your food without the danger of high-sodium levels in your body.

Tip #2: Spices and Herbs

No one likes tasteless meals which are why in general we add extra salt to our food. Since you need to lower your intake of salt to preserve your health, you can find healthier alternatives in herbs and spices that don't have high concentrations of sodium but will add taste to your food and make every meal delicious even without extra salt. We encourage you to experiment with different herbs and spices and find out which types of herbs are best suited to your taste. This way, your meals will taste great without the extra salt added during food processing.

Tip #3: Use Garlic and Ginger in Your Meals

To make up for the taste in unsalted food, you can use garlic and ginger. Besides from the fact that these will add more taste to your food, garlic and ginger also come with valuable health benefits and are good for your health as ginger represents a great antioxidant and garlic is known for having properties that are benevolent for your immune system.

Tip #4: Don't Use Salt and Pepper for Marinating Your Meat

Instead of marinating and softening the meat you eat with salt and pepper, you should switch to a healthier alternative and marinate your meat with a combination of garlic, herbs, honey, vinegar and olive oil. This marinade is low in sodium and it should make the meat tender and delicious if kept in the marinade for at least 30 minutes. It is recommended to keep the meat marinated in the fridge overnight.

Tip #5: Use More Fresh Products

Fresh food also has sodium concentrations as there are many ways in whi8ch sodium is introduced to our body and organism as a crucial mineral. However, fresh produce has far fewer sodium concentrations when compared to processed and canned foods. You should always choose fresh goods over-processed foods as processed food is rich in sodium and has added salt.

Incorporating Healthy Habits into Your Lifestyle

Kidneys are doing hard work to keep you healthy and keep your system free of waste, excess water and redundant minerals and leftovers chemicals and nutrients ingested through your everyday meals. When renal functions are not performing as supposed to, then some of that hard work needs to be taken over by yourself to live a healthy life and preserve your health. To do so, you will need to work on incorporating healthy habits into your existing lifestyle and start working on diminishing habits that are in no way good for your condition.

You have already started living healthier by expelling and limiting foods that are naturally rich in sodium and potassium and have added salt and sodium, which is a great start.

Maintaining a Healthy Weight

Maintaining a healthy weight is important for renal patients as frequent weight changes may further damage your kidneys and harm your health. You need to make sure that you are not overeating to make up for the fact that you are missing out on certain types of meals as you are restricted from some food groups that may additionally harm your condition and damage your renal functions. The best way of maintaining a healthy weight is to eat regularly and try having smaller meal portions with fewer calories while taking all the nutrients you need.

Eating regularly and establishing a routine with your meals is also recommended. When it comes to food preparation as mentioned earlier in the book, use cooking techniques that originally require less oil and fat for preparation. Your diet may be diverse; however, you need to take care of portions and avoid responding to food cravings and eating more than your body needs.

Watch Your Calorie Intake

Calories should be watched closely in terms of avoiding consuming empty calories – the kind that can give you the energy your body needs but that won't offer essential nutrients that your body needs. Empty calories are usually found in sweets, sugary beverages and snacks. Avoid munching on snacks and sweets and find healthier alternatives in fruit and vegetables, as these food groups will provide you with all essential nutrients and have fewer calories than processed food with added sugar or added sodium.

Don't Take Weight Supplements

Maintaining a healthy weight is important for your health and will help you live a normal life even when your renal system is giving you a hard time; however, you should never take an alternative in a shortcut, meaning that you shouldn't rely on weight supplements and weight loss products for helping you lose or maintain your weight. Weight supplements may impose more threat to your health by adding more toxins and waste to your organism. Since kidneys are sue to expel and eject that waste, in cases where that is not the case due to slow or damaged renal system, your kidney condition may become worse. That is why we do not recommend taking any supplements for weight loss, especially not weight loss products that have not been adequately tested under the general medical standard. Instead of taking a shortcut, you should focus on changing your lifestyle and eating healthier for best weight maintenance results.

No Over-the-Counter Pills and Medications

Common pain killers that are usually taken and bought over-the-counter and without a prescription, and used for diminishing or relieving pain, as well as anti-inflammatory drugs, raise the risk of getting a kidney's disease or have kidney's condition worsened if and when taken regularly. Avoid taking pain killers unless prescribed by your doctor otherwise. If in pain, talk to your physician or a doctor specialist about which medications are safe for you. Avoid taking any type of medications and pills that are no9t specifically prescribed for you and by your doctor as your condition will most certainly become worse as you will be placing extra pressure on your kidneys due to consumption of these medications.

Avoid Sweets and Sugar-packed Goods

Patients with diabetes represent a risk group for getting chronic kidney diseases as well, while the overall conditions of patients with kidney's condition may get worse with frequent consumption of sugar and processed foods with added sugar. Just as we recommend to cut on your salt consumption to avoid having increased level of sodium in your body and further complications caused by redundant sodium, it is likewise recommended to cut on your sugar intake as well. Sugar may cause diabetes if taken regularly and in large quantities, and should be avoided. You may use fruit as a way healthier alternative, but try to avoid high-potassium foods such as bananas.

Get Plenty of Sleep

Sleep deprivation may cause all kinds of health conditions that may cause further damage to the body. This is the case because we use sleep to help our cells renew and our body recover. Whenever we don't get enough sleep, we get tired, feel fatigued, our blood pressure is fluctuating, we are losing focus and are often unable to perform daily tasks we normally do. Not getting the sleep you need will also make your body more prone to all kinds of disease and illness, while it will make your entire body feel alarmed and stressed, which should further have a devastating effect on your renal health. Make sure to address your body's needs and get as much sleep as you need.

Eat Healthily

Eating healthy should be the centerpiece of your new lifestyle as healthy food improves health and has numerous benefits for our body as well as mind. When eating unhealthy food in the long run, we are introducing our body to lots of waste that our organism doesn't needs, which is where the role of kidneys and our renal functions comes as crucial for our well-being. In cases where renal function is weak, slow or failing in performance, waste introduced through an unhealthy diet is causing various damage to the body, furthermore bringing more damage to kidneys and renal system, that way creating a vicious circle where your health condition is only getting worse. Make sure to cut on fast food and snacks, junk food, processed food, sweets and food packed with salt and additives. Focus on fresh groceries and healthily prepared food.

Check Your Blood Pressure

Blood pressure is the cause of many serious health conditions and it also represents one of the main causes and symptoms of renal diseases. High blood pressure causes kidney damage and may harm your cardiovascular health and cause a heart attack. In case you have high blood pressure, you should cut on your sodium intake, while kidney patients are advised to lower their sodium intake at all costs that way preventing increased blood pressure that is more likely to be triggered by salt intake and consumption of bad fat and highly processed foods. Instead of salt, try using garlic and lemon for most of your meals. While garlic holds anti-inflammatory properties and acts benevolently on our immune system, garlic is also said to be able to lower your blood pressure. Make sure that you are checking your blood pressure with your doctor regularly to avoid further complications and more damage to your kidneys.

Check Your Blood Sugar

Diabetes, as mentioned earlier, can cause damage to kidneys where kidney's disease can even be triggered by diabetes. In cases where kidney's patients develop diabetes due to an improper diet or/and genetic predispositions, the overall condition of kidneys disease is set to worsen. That is why we recommend cutting on sugary treats and beverages, added sugar and processed foods. Preparing your food by yourself so that you can follow up on the amounts of sugar present in your everyday diet.

Lower Liquid Intake if Necessary

In some cases, patients suffering from a type of kidneys disease and who have slow or inefficient renal functions will be recommended by their doctor to cut on liquid intake, which usually includes drinking only water and in quantities less than a liter per day, where it is considered that a daily recommended dose of water consumption daily would be 2 liters. Unless stated otherwise, you can keep up with your normal tempo when it comes to liquid and water intake. However, you should note that since kidneys are due to release excess water from your body, in cases where the renal system is inefficient, redundant water won't be able to leave the body as kidneys would be struggling with liquid ejection. The retained excess water may cause damage to your heart and lungs, and cause more damage to your kidneys, while increased sodium encourages your body to keep more water than necessary at the same time causing dehydration and making you drink more liquids. Excess liquids are placing pressure on your kidneys, which is why it may be recommended to cut on liquid intake and only keep drinking enough water to keep you hydrated while lowering your sodium intake.

Quit Smoking!

Smoking may cause all kinds of cancer, stroke, heart attack and cardiovascular diseases, and it also increases chances for getting kidneys cancer. Patients who had already been diagnosed with a kidney's disease should stop smoking as inhaling of cigarette smoke may cause further damage to the kidneys because smoking slows down the flow of blood that runs through kidneys, that way disabling these vital organs from performing functions that are crucial for your health.

Cut Your Meat Meals

Meat is packed with protein and your kidneys are set to eject the leftover waste produced when our organism processes the protein and our muscles take what they need from nutrients introduced with meat. Meat is delicious and nutritious, yes, however, too much meat is surely set to mess with your health and will place more pressure on your kidneys. Processed protein creates waste that your body needs to get rid of, as mentioned before, this waste is called urea and creatinine and our body ejects it with the help of kidneys and through urine that way keeping us healthy and our body free of waste. To help improve your renal health, you may seek for meat substitution in salmon or start eating meat moderately and in smaller portions. A general recommendation would be twice to three times a week once a day for meat portions, while you should also make sure to cook your meat with less oil and no fat added. Make sure to choose meat pieces that have less fat and more lean meat. Cook or slow cook your meat with herbs and spices instead frying your meat and adding salt.

No Alcohol

Drinking is proven to have devastating effects on kidneys even at people who haven't been diagnosed with a form of kidney's disease, as frequent and excess alcohol consumption increases the risk of getting a type of chronic kidneys disease and brings extended damage to an already damaged renal system. Stay away from alcohol even if you feel tempted. Alcohol is another form of liquid that your kidneys need to process and take care off, alongside introducing toxins to your body that may cause inflammation. Sugary alcohol beverages additionally contribute to weight gain, which could consequently bring more damage to your kidneys.

Prepare Your Meals

The best way of knowing what you are consuming to the tiniest detail is to prepare your food by yourself, you may love take-outs and nights when you are having your dinner out, but try to prepare most of your food by yourself, including your snacks. When making your meals, make sure that the food you are using is mostly fresh and low in sodium, potassium and low concentrations of other nutrients that can be harmful to your renal health. Try to take your lunch from home when going to work instead of eating in a cafeteria or a restaurant. Focus on preparing meals by boiling, steaming, slow cooking or baking instead of using frying techniques.

No Added Salt and Processed Foods

Beside from encouraging more fresh groceries with low-sodium and low-potassium concentrations, we also encourage you to avoid adding salt to your meals as well as to follow up with food labels to make sure that you are nor consuming food that has high concentrations of sodium as well as potassium. Processed foods such as processed meat, boxed and packaged goods, snacks, junk food and fast food, sweets and cookies, candy and similar sugary treats are bad for you in general, and with added salt may additionally harm our kidneys and slow down your renal functions, that way damaging your kidneys as these vital organs are not able to process and level all the sodium in your body with the presence of chronic kidney disease.

Watch for Your Potassium Intake

Potassium is an otherwise essential mineral that your body needs, however, when present at increased levels in your body, it represents waste that damaged kidneys are not able to eject from your system, potentially causing hyperkalemia and cause more damage to your kidneys and an already damaged renal system. Follow up with the grocery list we have made on foods that are normally low in potassium concentrations so that your body may receive the quantity of this vital mineral it needs without struggling with excess waste. Be aware that some low-sodium products may have increased concentration of potassium. Consult your doctor on the matter of potassium and deliberate the average amount of potassium you may have on a weekly and daily basis with your condition.

Be Active and Exercise

Being active and exercising is important for everyone as your body needs activity to be able to burn calories that you are introducing to your body with every meal. Physical activity also encourages the production of serotonin – the happiness hormone – which makes you feel motivated and refreshed once healthy physical activity becomes a part of your routine. Physical condition is great for your health as well and should help you battle issues you are having with your renal health as well.

Chapter 10: Renal Diet And Lifestyle Guidance

1. Always follow your dietician's advice in conjunction with any research or cookbooks you use: During kidney disease, this is extremely important. They can advise you about sodium, phosphorous and potassium content of favorite foods and give you recommendations on how to reduce your sodium intake. Your diet will be tailored to you, taking into account the stage of kidney disease you're in and any other illnesses or diseases you suffer from.

2. Keep a Food Diary: You should track what you're eating and drinking to stay within the guidelines and recommendations given to you. Apps such as My Fitness Pal make this extremely easy and even track many of the minerals and levels in foods including sodium, protein etc. There are also apps specifically made for kidney disease patients to track sodium, phosphorous and potassium levels.

3. Read Food Labels: Some foods have hidden sodium in them, even if they don't taste salty. You will need to cut back on the amount of canned, frozen, and processed foods you eat. Check your beverages for added sodium.

Check food labels to avoid: Potassium chloride, Tetrasodium phosphate, Sodium phosphate, Trisodium phosphate, Tricalcium phosphate, Phosphoric acid, Polyphosphate, Hexametaphosphate, Pyrophosphate, Monocalcium phosphate, Dicalcium phosphate, Aluminum phosphate, Sodium tripolyphosphate, Sodium polyphosphate.

4. Flavor foods with fresh herbs and spices instead of shop-bought dressings and condiments: These add flavor and variety to your meals and are not packed with sodium; spices also have many health benefits! Also, stay away from salt substitutes and seasonings that contain potassium. Use citrus fruits and vinegar for dressings and to add flavor.

5: Keep Up Your Appointments With Your Doctor or Nephrologist:

Let your doctor know if you notice any swelling or changes in your weight.

6. Monitor drink and fluid intake: You have probably been told you need to drink up to eight glasses of water a day. This is true for a healthy body but people experiencing the later stages of CKD, these fluids can build up and cause additional problems. The restriction of fluids will differ from person to person. Things to take into consideration are swelling urine output and weight gain. Your weight will be recorded before dialysis begins and once it's over. This is done to determine how much fluid to remove from your body. If you are undergoing haemodialysis, this will be recorded approximately three times a week. If you are undergoing peritoneal dialysis, your weight is recorded every day. If there is a significant weight gain you may be drinking too many fluids.

7. Measure portion sizes -Moderating your portion sizes is essential. Use smaller cups, bowls, or plates to avoid giving yourself oversized portions.

Measure your food so you can keep an accurate record of how much you are eating:

The size of your fist is equal to 1 cup.

The palm of your hand is equal to 3 ounces.

The tip of your thumb is equivalent to 1 teaspoon.

A poker chip is equal to 1 tablespoon.

Substitution Tips:

- Use plain white flour instead of whole-wheat/whole-grain
- Use all-purpose flour instead of self-raising,
- Use Stevia instead of sugar,
- Use egg whites rather than whole eggs,
- Use almond rice or soy milk instead of cows milk.

8. Other Advice: Be careful when eating in restaurants -ask for dressings and condiments on the side and watch out for soups and cured meats.

Watch out for convenience foods that are high in sodium.

Prepare your meals and freeze them for later use.

Drain liquids from canned vegetables and fruits to help control potassium levels.

Foods to Avoid:

- Cured meats
- Bacon and ham
- Cold cuts
- Frozen dinners
- Salted nuts
- Canned beans with salt added
- Canned entrées
- Raisins
- Oranges
- Cantaloupe
- Pumpkin
- Potatoes
- Dried beans
- Tomatoes
- Yogurt
- Ice Cream
- Milk
- Nuts and seeds
- Salt substitutes
- Molasses
- Chocolate
- Bottled coffee drinks
- Non-dairy creamers
- Cereal bars

- Enhanced chicken and meat
- Sodas
- Iced teas
- Flavored waters
- Sardines
- Offal
- Processed meats
- Dried beans
- Nuts and nut butter
- Avocado
- Pizza
- Biscuits, pancakes, waffles
- Corn tortillas
- Whole grain crackers, bread, cereals
- Bran
- Beer, chocolate drinks, cola, milk-based coffee
- Cheese
- Salted Butter
- Coconut
- Solid shortening

High potassium fruits should be avoided. A serving of the following listed fruits has more than 250 mg of potassium:

- 5 dried prunes or ½ cup prune juice
- 1/8 of a honeydew melon
- ¼ cup dates
- ½ cup orange juice or 1 small orange
- 1 small nectarine no bigger than 2 inches across

These vegetables have more than 250 mg of potassium in each 1.2 cup serving.

- Fresh beets
- Winter squash
- Tomatoes, juice, or ¼ cup sauce
- Sweet potatoes
- Potatoes
- Okra and Brussel sprouts
- ¼ avocado or 1 whole artichoke

Foods To Enjoy:

Red bell peppers have low potassium but lots of flavor. They are also a good way to get folic acid, fiber, vitamin C, A, and B6. Red bell peppers also contain lycopene - an antioxidant that helps protect against cancer. A ½ cup serving contains 10 mg of phosphorus, 88 mg of potassium and 1 mg of sodium.

Cabbage contains phytochemicals - a chemical compound found in fruits and vegetables that helps break up free radicals. Phytochemicals are known to protect against cancer and help keep your heart healthy. Cabbage is high in vitamin C, K, B6, folic acid and fiber. A ½ cup serving contains just 9 mg of phosphorus, 60 mg potassium, and 6 mg sodium.

Cauliflower contains indoles, glucosinolates, and thiocyanates. These help the liver get rid of toxins that could damage cell membrane and DNA. A ½ cup serving of boiled cauliflower has 20 mg phosphorus, 88 mg potassium, 9 mg sodium.

Garlic helps reduce inflammation, keeps plaque from building on your teeth, and lowers cholesterol. Just one clove of garlic has 4 mg of phosphorus, 12 mg of potassium and 1 mg of sodium.

Onion contains quercetin an antioxidant that protects against cancers and helps heart disease. Onions contain chromium - a mineral that helps with protein, carbohydrate and fat metabolism. A ½ cup serving has 3 mg phosphorus, 116 mg potassium, and 3 mg sodium.

Apples prevent constipation, reduce cholesterol, reduce the risk of cancer, and protects against heart disease. Apples have anti-inflammatory compounds and are high in fiber. Just 1 medium apple with the skin on has no sodium, 158 mg of potassium and 10 mg of phosphorus.

Cranberries can keep you from getting a bladder infection because they prevent bacteria from sticking to the bladder wall. Cranberries can also help the stomach from creating the bacteria that causes ulcers thus promoting good GI health. Cranberries can also protect against heart disease and cancer. A ½ cup cranberry juice cocktail has 3 mg phosphorus, 22 mg potassium, 3 mg sodium. A ¼ cup of cranberry sauce has 6 mg phosphorus, 17 mg potassium, and 35 mg sodium. A ½ cup of dried cranberries has 5 mg phosphorus, 24 mg potassium, and 2 mg sodium.

Blueberries help reduce inflammation. Blueberries contain manganese, fiber, and vitamin C. They also help protect the brain from the effects of aging. A ½ cup of fresh blueberries has 7 mg phosphorus, 65 mg potassium, and 4 mg sodium.

Raspberries contain phytonutrient ellagic acid which helps reduce free radical cell damage. They are high in vitamin C, manganese, folate, and fibre. A ½ cup of raspberries has 7 mg phosphorus, 93 mg potassium, 0 mg sodium.

Strawberries are a good source of manganese, vitamin C, and fibre. They provide anti-inflammatory and anti-cancer compounds and help to protect the heart. A ½ cup or 13 mg phosphorus, 120 mg potassium, 1 mg sodium.

Cherries, when eaten daily, can help reduce inflammation. A ½ cup serving of fresh cherries has 15 mg phosphorus, 160 mg potassium, 0 mg sodium.

Red grapes protect against heart disease by reducing blood clots. They also help protect against inflammation and cancer. A ½ cup red grapes has 4 mg phosphorus, 88 mg potassium, 1 mg sodium.

Egg whites contain the highest quality protein and essential amino acids. 2 egg whites contain 10 mg phosphorus, 108 mg potassium, 110 mg sodium, and 7 grams protein.

Fish is a source of protein and anti-inflammatory fats known as omega-3s. Omega-3s help fight heart disease and cancer. It is recommended that you eat fish two times a week.

Olive oil helps fight against oxidation and inflammation. Virgin olive oils contain more antioxidants. 1 tablespoon olive oil serving contains less than 0 mg of phosphorus, less than an mg of potassium, and 1 mg of sodium.

Vitamins and minerals: Our bodies need vitamins to be able to function correctly. The best way to achieve this is to make sure you eat a well-rounded diet. However, if you have chronic kidney disease, you may not be able to get all the recommended vitamins through diet alone. Vitamins that are usually recommended by your renal dietitian are vitamin C, biotin, pantothenic acid, niacin, vitamin B12, B6, B2, B1, and folic acid. You must consult your doctor or dietician before starting to take vitamin supplements.

C4: EATING OUT AND SHOPPING ON A RENAL DIET

Advice for Dining Out

You don't have to miss out on your favorite restaurant or cuisines! Look out for small or half portions and ask your server for your foods to be cooked without extra salts, butter or sauces. Avoid fried foods and opt for grilled or poached instead.

If you know you are going out to eat, plan. Look at the restaurant's menu beforehand and decide what you will order to avoid anxiety or stress on the night! Use the food lists above to help you choose and don't feel bad about asking them to cater to your needs. Be sure to take your phosphorus binders, if they have been prescribed to you. Take them with your meal instead of waiting until you get home.

Advice for traveling

Whatever your travel plans, you will have to eat. If you plan, you should be able to make a meal plan with your renal dietitian. Tell your dietitian where you are going and what you expect to eat at your destination.

Remember to pack any prescriptions you may have such as phosphate binders.

If you are diabetic remember to keep carbohydrate intake to a minimum. Try not to eat sweets such as sweetened drinks, fruit juices, cakes, pies, and candy. Don't consume salty foods like chips, crackers, and pretzels. Also limit condiments such as soy sauce, salad dressing, and ketchup. Keep a check on your blood sugar daily.

If going on a road trip or camping, avoid processed meats. If at all possible, use fresh-cooked meats, low-sodium deli meats, unsalted chicken or tuna.

Choose unsalted pretzels or crackers instead of potato chips. Salty foods need to be avoided if you are on a fluid restricted diet.

Take along nutritional drinks formulated for kidney patients. These can always be used as a meal replacement if need be.

Remember to check labels for sodium content.

Do not consume dairy products unless they are allowed as part of your diet plan.

If you are going on a cruise, all those buffet foods are tempting to eat 24 hours a day. To help with this predicament try to select fruits, salads, and vegetables from the lists above.

Remember to include a good source of protein with every meal and avoid bread and sauces that are salty. You could pack your snacks to eat between meals.

- Let the cruise line know of your dietary needs, most are willing to prepare special foods for you. Low-sodium meal options may also be available.
- If you are going to be traveling abroad and don't speak the language, bring a phrasebook that has a unit for ordering food.

Cooking Tips

- Grill, poach, roast or sauté meats instead of frying.
- Steam or boil vegetables instead of frying.
- Use healthy oils such as extra virgin olive oil to shallow fry.
- Soak fruit and vegetables in warm water for 2 hours before cooking to reduce potassium levels – especially potatoes!

- When using canned beans and vegetables, make sure to rinse and drain them.
- Drain liquid from canned or frozen vegetables and fruits.

One Last Thing:

Always remember to use new recipes and ingredients after speaking to your doctor or dietician; your needs will be unique to you depending on the stage of Chronic Kidney Disease you're experiencing. We hope that with your doctor's advice, along with our guidance and recipes that you can continue to enjoy cooking, eating and sharing meal times with your love ones.

All the best and happy cooking!

Conclusion

On the off chance that you are experiencing a renal issue, for example, kidney stones, at that point you might be intrigued to realize that a kidney diet has a noteworthy impact in alleviating unfavorable side effects and helping the kidney recuperate rapidly from the issue. While a few nourishments might be nutritious and useful for the body, they may present significant issues to the kidneys over the long haul. Along these lines, it is well-encouraged to eat suppers with some restraint and assessing the appropriateness of the eating regimen to your condition.

A kidney diet ought to maintain a strategic distance from calcium and phosphorous improved nourishments

Best case scenario, dietary changes, for example, evasion of calcium and phosphorous rich nourishments will become essential if certain kidney issues are at basic organizing. This applies generally to people who are in danger of building up a renal issue. The following are a portion of the dos and don'ts that you ought to think about when arranging your kidney diet.

Don'ts of a kidney diet

- Don't utilize nourishment plans in your eating routine for renal infection which have generous amounts of mineral salts particularly oxalate salts from calcium, phosphorus, manganese. These mineral components can cause quicker kidney degeneration and extreme weakness in kidney working.
- Don't eat overabundance segments of nourishments that have high convergences of immersed fats, for example, fries, burgers, and red meat or any handled food sources.
- Don't drink liquor, caffeinated beverages, or refreshments with high sugar content-both may exhaust the liver and intensify or cause degeneration of the kidney issue.

- Don't devour sugary substances, for example, tidbits, deserts, or confections since they cause a lack of hydration and exhaust the kidney simply like salts.
- Do not take a wide range of common red meat in your kidney diet-hamburger, pork, bacon, or lamb and their options seared, restored, or prepared meats, rather search for lean white meat from poultry.
- Do not utilize any fake sugars while planning nourishments since they have no healthful advantages
- Do not utilize margarine or mayonnaise yet options, for example, an avocado natural product on the off chance that you need to devour fat.
- Do not eat a bigger number of helpings than should be expected particularly to delights, for example, fries, frozen yogurts, soft drinks, and other sweet nourishments and a wide range of handled or canned nourishments
- Don't devour a greater number of starches than should be expected in your kidney diet and this incorporates such carbs like pasta, white rice, scones, white sugar, white rice, and pasta.

Do's of a kidney diet

- Do take enough liquids to keep centralization of minerals, for example, calcium and sodium on the kidney low. These will to guarantee appropriate kidney working, counteract lack of hydration which is the regular reason for kidney stones in the renal cylinders, and detoxify the kidney also.
- Do embrace a reasonable eating regimen for a renal illness which contains crisp vegetables, entire grains, and lean meat just as water. Greens and natural products plentiful in nutrients improve cell digestion and the working of organs.
- Do take fiber or fuse fiber-rich suppers and entire grains in your renal eating routine which are low in carbs however advance general wellbeing and lift kidney working.
- Do eat modestly and create smart dieting propensities to guarantee that your body gets the correct stock of minerals and supplements.

- Do eat vegetables and organic products as regularly as you can and consolidate them in your kidney diet intend to help your invulnerability and cell digestion

- Do utilize low-fat milk items, for example, milk powder on the off chance that you need to utilize them as opposed to utilizing milk with cream or fat.

- Do utilize monounsaturated fat or normal fat when cooking and lower the measure of fat that you expend every day in your dinners.

- Do grasp dynamic and energetic life to decrease heftiness or strange weight, help working of renal eating routine, and advance great body digestion and kidney working. Exercise guarantees blood dissemination to kidney and lifts exercises, for example, detoxification and separating.

CPSIA information can be obtained
at www.ICGtesting.com
Printed in the USA
LVHW100829181120
672011LV00010B/378